Applied Multilevel Analysis

A Practical Guide

This is a practical introduction to multilevel analysis suitable for all those doing research. Most books on multilevel analysis are written by statisticians, and they focus on the mathematical background. These books are difficult for non-mathematical researchers. In contrast, this volume provides an accessible account on the application of multilevel analysis in research. It addresses the practical issues that confront those undertaking research and wanting to find the correct answers to research questions. This book is written for non-mathematical researchers and it explains when and how to use multilevel analysis. Many worked examples, with computer output, are given to illustrate and explain this subject. Datasets of the examples are available on the Internet, so the reader can reanalyse the data. This approach will help to bridge the conceptual and communication gap that exists between those undertaking research and statisticians.

Practical Guides to Biostatistics and Epidemiology

Series advisors

Susan Ellenberg, *University of Pennsylvania School of Medicine*
Robert C. Elston, *Case Western Reserve University School of Medicine*
Brian Everitt, *Institute for Psychiatry, King's College London*
Frank Harrell, *Vanderbilt University Medical Centre Tennessee*
Jos W.R. Twisk, *Vrije Universiteit Medical Centre, Amsterdam*

This will be a series of short and practical but authoritative books for biomedical researchers, clinical investigators, public health researchers, epidemiologists, and non-academic and consulting biostatisticians who work with data from biomedical and epidemiological and genetic studies. Some books will be explorations of a modern statistical method and its application, others may focus on a particular disease or condition and the statistical techniques most commonly used in studying it.

This series is for people who use statistics to answer specific research questions. Books will explain the application of techniques, specifically the use of computational tools, and emphasize the interpretation of results, not the underlying mathematical and statistical theory.

Published in the series
Applied Multilevel Analysis, by **Jos W.R. Twisk**

Applied Multilevel Analysis

A Practical Guide

Jos W. R. Twisk
Vrije Universiteit Medical Centre, Amsterdam

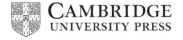

CAMBRIDGE
UNIVERSITY PRESS

CAMBRIDGE UNIVERSITY PRESS
Cambridge, New York, Melbourne, Madrid, Cape Town, Singapore, São Paulo

CAMBRIDGE UNIVERSITY PRESS
The Edinburgh Building, Cambridge CB2 2RU, UK
Published in the United States of America by Cambridge University Press,
New York

www.cambridge.org
Information on this title: www.cambridge.org/9780521849753

© J.W.R. Twisk 2006

First published 2006

Printed in the United Kingdom at the University Press, Cambridge

A catalogue record for this publication is available from the British Library

Library of Congress Cataloguing in Publication data

ISBN 13 978 0 521 84975 3 hardback
ISBN 10 0 521 84975 6 hardback
ISBN 13 978 0 521 61498 6 paperback
ISBN 10 0 521 61498 8 paperback

'I've seen this happen in other people's lives
and now it's happening in mine' MORRISSEY, THE SMITHS

To Marjon, Mike, and Nick

Contents

Preface

The topic of this book is multilevel analysis but, although this is a mathematical topic, it has been written by an epidemiologist. This could, perhaps, be a disadvantage, because the mathematical background of multilevel analysis will not be discussed in detail. However, it can also be seen as an advantage, because it implies that the emphasis of this book lies more on the application of multilevel analysis. Many books have been written on multilevel analysis, but most (all) of them have been written by statisticians, and therefore they mainly focus on the mathematical background of multilevel analysis. The problem with that approach is that such books are very difficult for non-mathematical researchers to understand. And yet, these non-mathematical researchers are expected to use multilevel analysis to analyse their data. In fact, a researcher is not primarily interested in the basic (difficult) mathematical background of the statistical methods, but in finding correct answers to research questions. Furthermore, researchers want to know how to apply a statistical technique and how to interpret the results. Due to their different basic interests and different levels of thinking, communication problems between statisticians and epidemiologists are quite common, and they often communicate on different levels. This, in addition to the growing interest in multilevel analysis, initiated the writing of this book. This book is written for 'non-statistical' researchers, and it aims to provide a practical guide as to when and how to use multilevel analysis. The purpose of this book is to build a bridge between the different communication levels that exist between statisticians and researchers when addressing the topic of multilevel analysis.

Jos Twisk

Amsterdam, April 2005

Acknowledgements

I am very grateful to all my colleagues and students who came to me with (mostly) practical questions on multilevel analysis. This book is based on all those questions. Furthermore, I would like to thank Bernard Uitdehaag, Dirk Knol, and Hans Berkhof who critically read preliminary drafts of some chapters and provided very helpful comments. In addition I would like to thank Faith Maddever who corrected the English language.

Amsterdam, April 2005

1

Introduction

1.1 Introduction

The popularity of applying multilevel analysis has increased rapidly over the past 10 years. A very small non-systematic search in 'pubmed' showed that in 1995, 22 papers were published in which multilevel analysis was applied. In 2000 this number increased to 86, while in 2004 the number of papers in which multilevel analysis was applied rose to over 170. Figure 1.1 shows the development from 1995 to 2004 in the number of published papers in which multilevel analysis was applied.

The literature on multilevel analysis is somewhat confusing, because multilevel analysis or multilevel modelling is also referred to as hierarchical

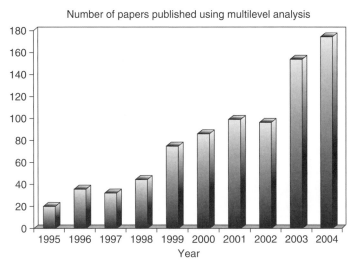

Figure 1.1. Development from 1995 to 2004 in the number of published papers in which multilevel analysis was applied.

modelling, mixed effect analysis/modelling or random effects analysis/ modelling. However, in most situations all these different terms are exactly the same.

1.2 Background of multilevel analysis

Multilevel analysis was first developed for educational research (Goldstein, 1987; Goldstein and Cuttance, 1988; Nuttall et al., 1989; Woodhouse and Goldstein, 1989; Plewis, 1991; Goldstein, 1992). Analysing the performance of students, the researchers realised that the observations of students in the same class were not independent of each other. Because 'standard' statistical tools assume independent observations, it is not really appropriate to use these 'standard' statistical tools to analyse the performance of students. The students in the same class can be described as a sort of hierarchy; students are clustered within classes (see Figure 1.2). This situation is known as a two-level data structure, the first level being the students and the second level being the classes. The general idea of multilevel analysis is that this hierarchy is taken into account in the analysis, or in other words, it takes into account the dependency of the observations. Within the educational setting, we can go one step further (or perhaps we should say one step higher), because not only the students are clustered within classes, but the classes are also clustered within schools (see Figure 1.3). This situation is referred to as a three-level data structure, the students being level 1, the classes being

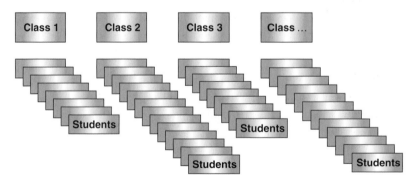

Figure 1.2.   Illustration of a two-level hierarchical data structure. Observations of students are clustered within classes.

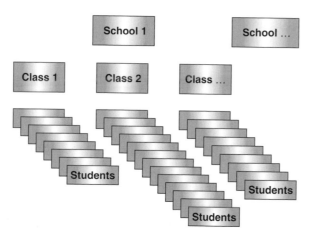

Figure 1.3. Illustration of a three-level hierarchical data structure. Observations of students are clustered within classes and the observations of classes are clustered within schools.

level 2, and the schools being level 3. Again, the general idea of multilevel analysis in this situation is that it takes into account the dependency of observations, not only within classes, but also within schools.

1.3 General approach

Although there is a considerable amount of literature on multilevel analysis, most of it is characterised by a mathematical approach (Bryk and Raudenbush, 1992; Goldstein, 1995; Hox, 1995; Kreft and De Leeuw, 1998; Snijders and Boschker, 1999; Little et al., 2000; McCullagh and Searle, 2001; Raudenbush and Hox, 2002; Bryk, 2002; Goldstein, 2003; Reise and Duan, 2003). This book will follow a more practical approach, which will make it (hopefully) easier to read and more understandable for non-mathematical readers. A review of the literature identified only a few other papers that tried to follow a more practical approach (see for instance, Korff et al., 1992; Rice and Leyland, 1996; Greenland, 2000a; Greenland, 2000b; Livert et al., 2001; Diez Roux, 2002; Leyland and Groenewegen, 2003; Merlo, 2003). Furthermore, the emphasis of this book will lie on the interpretation of the results of multilevel analysis, on the research questions that can be answered with multilevel analysis, and on the differences between multilevel analysis and the so-called 'naive' approaches that do not take into account the dependency of observations. Therefore, in each chapter, the (mathematically difficult) statistical analyses will be explained by using relatively simple examples, accompanied by computer output.

1.4 Prior knowledge

In this book an attempt has been made to keep the complicated statistical techniques as simple as possible. The basis of the explanations will be the underlying research question and the interpretation of the results of the statistical analysis. However, it will be assumed that the reader has some prior knowledge about 'standard' statistical regression techniques, such as linear regression analysis, logistic regression analysis, multinomial logistic regression analysis, and Poisson regression analysis. This is necessary, because multilevel analysis can be seen as an extension of the 'standard' regression techniques. So, multilevel analysis with a continuous outcome variable is an extension of linear regression analysis, multilevel analysis with a dichotomous outcome variable is an extension of logistic regression analysis, and so on.

1.5 Example datasets

All datasets that will be used in the examples will be available from the internet (http:\www.emgo.nl\researchtools), and can be reanalysed by the reader. This will certainly improve understanding of the general theories underlying multilevel analysis.

In general, the research question to be answered in (almost) all examples is more or less the same: What is the relationship between total cholesterol and age? This relationship will be analysed in many different ways to demonstrate the various possibilities of multilevel analysis. The outcome variable total cholesterol will be divided into two groups to illustrate multilevel analysis with dichotomous outcome variables (i.e. logistic multilevel analysis), and total cholesterol will be divided into three groups to illustrate multilevel analysis with a categorical outcome variable (i.e. multinomial multilevel analysis).

1.6 Software

All the analysis in the first part of the book (up to Chapter 9) are performed with multilevel analysis for Windows (MLwiN) (version 1.1 and version 2.0; Goldstein et al., 1998; Rasbash et al., 1999; Rashbash et al., 2003). In Chapter 9 a comparison will be made between various software packages that are (more or less) suitable for multilevel analysis. This comparison includes the following software packages: SPSS (version 12; Wolfinger et al., 1994; Landau and Everitt, 2004), STATA (version 7; Stata Corporation, 1999; Stata Reference Manual, 2001), SAS (version 8; Littel et al., 1991; Littel et al., 1996), and R (R Development Core Team, 2004). Both syntax and output will accompany the overview of the different packages. For detailed information about the different software packages, reference is made to the software manuals.

Basic principles of multilevel analysis

2.1 Introduction

To explain the basic principles of multilevel analysis, the application of multi-level analysis on a continuous outcome variable will first be discussed (i.e. linear multilevel analysis). The most important basic principle to be considered is the fact that linear multilevel analysis can be seen as an extended linear regression analysis. So, to understand the basic principles of multi-level analysis, linear regression analysis must be the starting point. Suppose that we are performing a study to investigate the relationship between total cholesterol and age. Figure 2.1 shows the results of this linear regression analysis and Equation (2.1) describes the linear regression model.

$$\text{Total cholesterol} = \beta_0 + \beta_1 \times \text{age} + \varepsilon \tag{2.1}$$

where total cholesterol = outcome variable; β_0 = intercept; β_1 = regression coefficient for age; age = independent variable, and ε = error/residual.

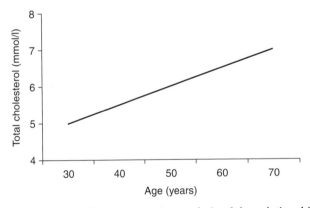

Figure 2.1. Illustration of a linear regression analysis of the relationship between total cholesterol and age.

The interpretation of the regression coefficients of this linear regression analysis is very straightforward. The intercept (β_0) is the value of the outcome variable (total cholesterol) when the independent variable (age) is zero. The regression coefficient for age (β_1) reflects the difference in total cholesterol for subjects who differ 1 year in age. Suppose now that we want to correct the analysis for gender. Males are different from females, and therefore we want to correct for gender (Equation (2.2)).

$$\text{Total cholesterol} = \beta_0 + \beta_1 \times \text{age} + \beta_2 \times \text{gender} + \varepsilon \qquad (2.2)$$

where β_2 = regression coefficient for gender.

Suppose that males are coded as 0 and females are coded as 1. The intercept β_0 reflects the intercept for males, while $\beta_0 + \beta_2$ reflects the intercept for females. So a correction for gender actually means that the intercept of the regression line is assumed to be different for males and females (see Figure 2.2).

We can go one step further. In the study population there are several patients who 'belong' to the same medical doctor. It is very reasonable to assume that the characteristics of a population of patients 'belonging' to a particular medical doctor differ from those of the population of patients 'belonging' to another medical doctor. These differences can, for instance, be caused by the area in which the medical doctor is practising, by certain personality characteristics of the medical doctor, etc. Anyway, because of this,

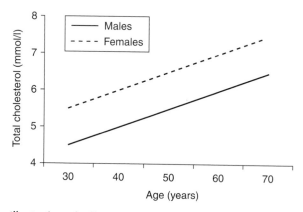

Figure 2.2. Illustration of a linear regression analysis of the relationship between total cholesterol and age, corrected for gender.

we want to correct for medical doctor in the linear regression analysis. Again, a correction for medical doctor actually means that different intercepts are estimated for each medical doctor (see Figure 2.3).

However, when a correction is made for medical doctor, a problem arises, because the medical doctor variable is not a continuous one, and when there are more than two medical doctors involved in the study the medical doctor variable is also not a dichotomous one. The medical doctor variable is a categorical variable (more specifically a nominal variable), and when a correction is made for a categorical variable, such as medical doctor, it means that dummy variables have to be created. The number of dummy variables depends on the number of medical doctors involved in the study (i.e. the number of medical doctors minus 1), and for all those dummy variables separate regression coefficients must be estimated (Equation (2.3)).

$$\text{Total cholesterol} = \beta_0 + \beta_1 \times \text{age} + \beta_2 \times \text{dummyMD}_1$$
$$+ \beta_3 \times \text{dummyMD}_2 + \dots + \beta_m$$
$$\times \text{dummyMD}_{m-1} + \varepsilon \tag{2.3}$$

where β_2 till β_m = regression coefficients for the dummy variables representing the different medical doctors, and m = number of medical doctors.

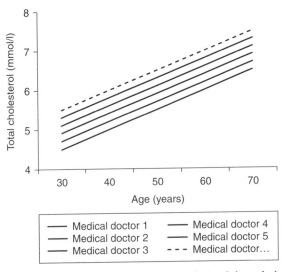

Figure 2.3. Illustration of a linear regression analysis of the relationship between total cholesterol and age, corrected for medical doctor.

So, if there are 12 medical doctors involved in the study, 11 additional regression coefficients must be estimated in the linear regression analysis. This is a 'dramatic' waste of power and efficiency, because the medical doctor variable was only added to the regression analysis to be corrected for, and there is no real interest in the different cholesterol values for each of the separate medical doctors. A much more powerful and efficient way to correct for medical doctor is provided by multilevel analysis. By using multilevel analysis, not all separate intercepts are estimated, but the variance of the intercepts is estimated. So, instead of estimating 11 intercepts, only one variance parameter is estimated. The estimation of the variance of the intercepts is also referred to as 'assuming or allowing the intercepts to be random', i.e. a random intercept. Therefore, multilevel analysis is also known as random coefficient analysis.

In multilevel terminology it is said that the observations that are made of the patients are 'clustered within medical doctors'. The observations of patients within one medical doctor are correlated, and therefore a correction must be made for medical doctor. Because of this clustering, it is also said that there is a two-level structure in the data. The observations of the patients are the lower level, while the medical doctor is the higher level (see Figure 2.4). Again, due to the fact that lower and higher levels exist in the data, multilevel analysis or multilevel modelling is also referred to as hierarchical modelling.

So, in general, multilevel analysis is a very efficient way of correcting for a categorical variable with many categories. Of course, there is some sort of trade-off. This trade-off is the assumption that the different intercepts for the different medical doctors are normally distributed. So, when performing

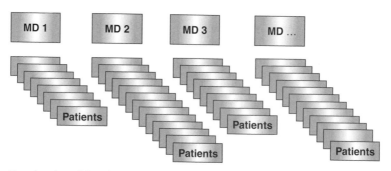

Figure 2.4. Two-level multilevel structure; patients are clustered within medical doctors.

a multilevel analysis, it is important to realise that this 'normality' assumption underlies the estimation procedure (see Section 2.7).

2.2 Example

The example that will be used to explain the basic principles of multilevel analysis is a very simple one: a cross-sectional study investigating the relationship between serum cholesterol and age. In this study, different medical doctors are involved, or in other words, the observations of the patients are clustered within medical doctors.

Output 2.1 shows the MLwiN output of the dataset used in this example.

Output 2.1. Descriptive information regarding the example dataset

1	total cholester(			Refresh	Categories	? Help		
	Name		**n**	**missing**	**min**		**max**	
1	total cholesterol		441	0	3,9		8,86	
2	medical doctor		441	0	1		12	
3	age		441	0	44		86	
4	id		441	0	1		441	
5	cons		441	0	1		1	

From Output 2.1 it can be seen that there are 441 patients with an age range of 44–86 years. Serum cholesterol levels range from 3.90 mmol/l to 8.86 mmol/l. Furthermore, it can be seen that there are 12 medical doctors involved in the study. In addition to these variables, there is also a variable named *cons*, with 441 observations ranging between 1 and 1. This variable is thus a row of only ones, and it is necessary in MLwiN to estimate an intercept of the regression line. Output 2.2 shows the results of the regression analysis without correcting for medical doctor. This kind of analysis is also referred to as 'naive' regression analysis, because it ignores the possible clustering of data, i.e. it ignores the fact that the observations of patients within the same medical doctor are correlated.

Output 2.2. Results of a 'naive' analysis of the relationship between total cholesterol and age

---

```
total cholesterol_ij ~ N(XB, Ω)
total cholesterol_ij = β_0i cons + 0,0513(0,0043)age_ij
β_0i = 2,7987(0,2680) + e_0ij

[e_0ij] ~ N(0, Ω_e) : Ω_e = [0,6961(0,0469)]

-2*loglikelihood(IGLS) = 1091,7520(441 of 441 cases in use)
```

The first line of Output 2.2 shows that total cholesterol is the outcome variable and that this outcome variable is assumed to follow a normal distribution. It can also be seen that there are two levels considered (subscripts i and j are indicators of the two levels), and although a 'naive' analysis is performed, in MLwiN the levels in the dataset should already be defined, because otherwise no analyses can be performed. The lower level (i) is the patient and the higher level (j) is the medical doctor (the observations of the patients are clustered within the medical doctors). The second line of the output shows the regression equation. From this regression equation it can be seen that a difference of 1 year in age is associated with a difference of 0.0513 mmol/l in total cholesterol. The value between brackets (i.e. 0.0043) is the standard error of the regression coefficient, and can be used to evaluate the significance of the relationship between age and total cholesterol. This is done with the Wald test, which involves dividing the regression coefficient by its standard error. This quantity squared is called the Wald statistic. The Wald statistic follows a Chi-square distribution, with one degree of freedom. In this example the Wald statistic is $(0.0513/0.0043)^2 = 142.3$, which is highly significant. It should be noted that the Chi-square distribution with one degree of freedom is the same as the standard normal distribution squared. This means that the same p-value can be derived by dividing the regression coefficient by its standard error, which then follows a standard normal distribution. The standard error can also be used to create a 95% confidence interval (CI) around the regression coefficient. This can be done in the 'traditional' way by taking the regression coefficient ± 1.96 times the standard error. In this example the 95% CI ranges from 0.0429 to 0.0597.

The third line of the output shows the value of the intercept. As was already mentioned earlier, *cons* is a row of ones, and therefore β_0 can be interpreted as the intercept. It can also be seen that the intercept has only one subscript i. This means that there is only variation on the individual level. This variation on the individual level is the overall 'error' variance, 'residual' variance or 'unexplained' variance (e_{0ij}). The value of the intercept is 2.7987 and, as for 'standard' linear regression analysis, this is the estimated total cholesterol value for the situation in which all determinants in the regression model have the value of zero. In this simple example, the value of the intercept can be interpreted as the value of total cholesterol when age = 0. The standard error for the intercept is also shown, and this can be used to test whether or not the intercept differs significantly from zero, but this is usually not of interest. The fourth line of the output shows the magnitude of the 'error variance' (e_{0ij}) and its corresponding standard error. Although the 'naive' analysis is basically a 'standard' linear regression analysis, the difference between a 'standard' linear regression analysis and the same analysis performed with MLwiN is that the regression coefficients in the latter are estimated by maximum likelihood, while the regression coefficients in 'standard' linear regression analysis are estimated with ordinary least squares (OLS). From the maximum likelihood estimation procedure, a log likelihood can be obtained. The -2 log likelihood is shown in the last line of the output (i.e. 1091.7520). The absolute value of the -2 log likelihood is hardly informative, but the value will be used in the likelihood ratio test in order to evaluate whether or not random regression coefficients must be considered. This will be explained in the following part of this section.

In the second step of the example analysis, a correction is made for medical doctor. As mentioned before, this is done by estimating the variance of the intercepts for the different medical doctors. Output 2.3 shows the result of this analysis.

In the second line of Output 2.3 it can be seen that a subscript j is added to the intercept, which indicates that a random intercept is allowed. Note that the subscript j refers to the highest level, i.e. the medical doctor. So, in other words, the subscript j means that a correction for medical doctor is added to the model. Compared to Output 2.2, in the third line of Output 2.3 it can be seen that the intercept consist of the actual value of the intercept, an error variance (e_{0ij}) and a new component which reflects the variance in

Output 2.3. Results of a linear multilevel analysis of the relationship between total cholesterol and age, with a random intercept at the medical doctor level

```
total cholesterol_ij ~ N(XB, Ω)
total cholesterol_ij = β_0ij cons + 0,0496(0,0031)age_ij
β_0ij = 2,9058(0,2591) + u_0j + e_0ij

[u_0j] ~ N(0, Ω_u) : Ω_u = [0,3686(0,1542)]
[e_0ij] ~ N(0, Ω_e) : Ω_e = [0,3315(0,0226)]

-2*loglikelihood(IGLS) = 809,3788(441 of 441 cases in use)
```

the intercepts of the different medical doctors (u_{0j}). The magnitude of this variance (and the corresponding standard error) is shown in the fourth line of the output. In this particular example the variance is 0.3686. The fifth line of the output shows the error variance. If this error variance is compared to the error variance in Output 2.2 (the model without a random intercept, i.e. without correcting for medical doctor) it can be seen that in the second analysis the error variance is highly reduced. In fact, most of the error variance from the 'naive' analysis is 'explained' by adding the random intercept to the model, i.e. most of the error variance is 'explained' by adding the medical doctor variable to the model. The question that then arises is whether or not it is necessary to correct for medical doctor or not; or, in other words, whether or not it is necessary to allow the intercepts to differ between the medical doctors. This question can be answered by performing the likelihood ratio test. The likelihood ratio test compares the -2 log likelihood of the model with a random intercept and the -2 log likelihood of the model without a random intercept. The difference between the -2 log likelihoods of the two models follows a Chi-square distribution. The number of degrees of freedom for this Chi-square distribution is equal to the difference in the number of parameters to be estimated in the two models. In the present example the difference between the two -2 log likelihoods is: 1091.7520 − 809.3788 = 282.3732. This difference follows a Chi-square distribution with one degree of freedom, because compared to the 'naive' analysis, in the second analysis only the variance of the intercepts is additionally estimated. This difference is highly significant. It is argued that when variance parameters are added to the model, the difference between the two $-2\log$ likelihoods should be tested one-sided, because a variance can only be positive, and therefore the difference between the $-2\log$ likelihoods can only be in one direction (Goldstein, 1995; Lin, 1997; Goldstein, 2003). It is rather strange that for the likelihood ratio test in multilevel analysis one-sided p-values are used, while for likelihood ratio tests in 'standard' logistic or Cox-regression analysis, for instance two-sided p-values are always used. In these 'standard' situations basically the same phenomenon occurs, because adding variables to models can only lead to a $-2\log$ likelihood change in one direction. Although in practice it is not really a big deal whether one-sided or two-sided p-values are used, it is important to realise that this contradiction exists in the literature.

The most interesting information in the output is still the second line, which shows the regression coefficient for age. Corrected for medical doctor, the regression coefficient decreased slightly from 0.0513 to 0.0496. So, a difference of 1 year in age between patients is associated with a difference of 0.0496 mmol/l in total cholesterol. When the Wald test is performed for this regression coefficient, it is obvious that there is still a highly significant relationship between age and total cholesterol. The Wald statistic is $(0.0496/0.0031)^2 = 256$ and according to the Chi-square distribution with one degree of freedom, this is highly significant. When reporting the result of this analysis, the regression coefficient and the 95% CI are usually presented. Again, the 95% CI can be estimated by applying the equation: regression coefficient ± 1.96 times the standard error. In the present example the 95% CI around the regression coefficient of 0.0496 ranges from 0.0435 to 0.0557.

2.3 Intraclass correlation coefficient

Based on the variance of intercepts and the remaining error variance, the so-called intraclass correlation coefficient (ICC) can be estimated. This ICC is an indication of the correlation of the observations of the patients belonging to the same medical doctor, i.e. it is an indication of the dependency of the patient observations within the medical doctors. The ICC is defined as the variance between medical doctors divided by the total variance, where the total variance is defined as the summation of the variance between medical doctors and the variance within medical doctors. Although some people find it counter-intuitive, the smaller the variance within the medical doctors, the greater the ICC. Figures 2.5a–d illustrate this phenomenon. Figure 2.5a shows the distribution of a particular outcome variable, and in Figures 2.5b–d, the outcome variable is divided into three groups (e.g. the observations belong to three different medical doctors). In Figure 2.5b, the

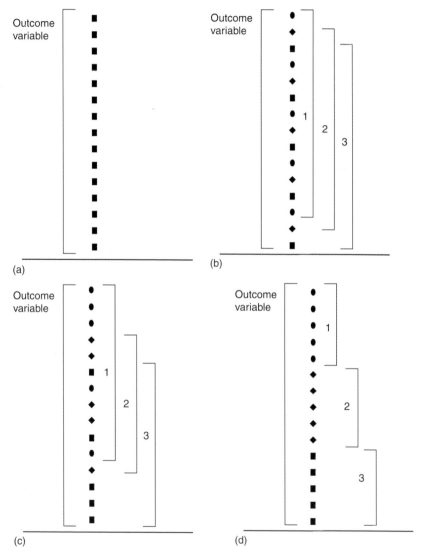

Figure 2.5 (a–d). Illustration of the intraclass correlation coefficient (ICC). The higher the variance within the groups, the lower the ICC.

ICC is low, because the variance within groups is rather high and the variance between groups is rather low. In Figure 2.5c the groups are more spread out, and therefore the between group variance increases and the within group variance decreases. As a consequence, the ICC is increased. In Figure 2.5d the difference between the groups is maximal. In other words, the within group variance is minimised and the between group variance is maximised. Therefore, in the last situation, the ICC is the greatest.

Going back to the results of the example given in Output 2.3, the ICC can be calculated by dividing the between medical doctor variance (i.e. 0.3686) by the total variance, which is calculated by summation of the between medical doctor variance and the within medical doctor variance (i.e. 0.3686 + 0.3315). So, in this example the ICC is: 0.3686/0.7001 = 0.526. It should be noted that in 'real life' cross-sectional studies in general the ICC's are much lower than in the present example. In most 'real life' cross-sectional studies the ICC will not be higher than 0.20. The reason for this relatively high ICC is that the example dataset is slightly manipulated and is purely for educational purposes.

2.4 Random slopes

Up to now, we have only considered a situation in which the intercept of the regression model is allowed to differ between groups. Let us go back to the regression model in which we wanted to analyse the relationship between total cholesterol and age, corrected for gender (Equation (2.2)).

Suppose now that it is not only assumed that the intercepts are different for males and females, but that the relationship between total cholesterol and age is also different for males and females. To allow for that, an interaction term between gender and age must be added to the regression model (Equation (2.4)). By adding an interaction between age and gender to the regression model, different 'slopes' of the regression line are estimated for males and females (see Figure 2.6).

$$\text{Total cholesterol} = \beta_0 + \beta_1 \times \text{age} + \beta_2 \times \text{gender}$$
$$+ \beta_3 \times (\text{age} \times \text{gender}) + \varepsilon \qquad (2.4)$$

where β_3 = regression coefficient for the interaction between gender and age.

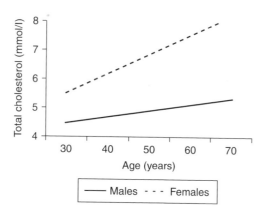

Figure 2.6. Illustration of a linear regression analysis of the relationship between total cholesterol and age, with an interaction between gender and age.

When the possible effect modifier (i.e. gender) is a dichotomous variable, just one interaction term has to be added to the regression model. However, when it is not the interaction with gender that is of interest, but the interaction with medical doctor, the same problems that were described before arise. So, when the observations are clustered within medical doctors, it may be reasonable to assume that the relationship between age and total cholesterol is different for different medical doctors. In other words, in this situation different 'slopes' of the regression line have to be estimated for each medical doctor (see Figure 2.7).

In a 'standard' regression analysis this can be done by adding interaction terms between age and the dummy variables representing the different medical doctors to the regression model (Equation (2.5)).

$$
\begin{aligned}
\text{Total cholesterol} = {} & \beta_0 + \beta_1 \times \text{age} + \beta_2 \times \text{dummyMD}_1 \\
& + \ldots + \beta_m \times \text{dummyMD}_{m-1} + \beta_{m+1} \\
& \times (\text{dummyMD}_1 \times \text{age}) + \ldots + \beta_{2m-1} \\
& \times (\text{dummyMD}_{m-1} \times \text{age}) + \varepsilon
\end{aligned} \tag{2.5}
$$

where β_{m+1} till β_{2m-1} = regression coefficients for the interactions between the dummy variables representing the different medical doctors and age, and m = number of medical doctors.

In our example with 12 medical doctors, this will mean that 11 interaction terms have to be added to the regression model. Estimating 11 regression

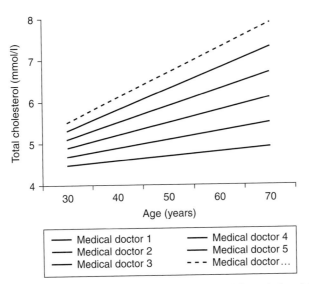

Figure 2.7. Illustration of a linear regression analysis of the relationship between total cholesterol and age, with an interaction between medical doctor and age.

coefficients that are not of major interest will (again) lead to a(n) (enormous) loss of power and efficiency. Comparable to what has been described for the different intercepts, we are still only interested in the overall relationship between age and total cholesterol. To cope with this, also for this situation multilevel analysis provides a very efficient solution. As for the different intercepts, one variance parameter can also be estimated for the different slopes of the regression lines (reflecting the relationship between age and total cholesterol) for the different medical doctors. So, in addition to 'random intercepts', 'random slopes' can also be considered.

2.5 Example

Let us go back to the example dataset that was described in Section 2.2 to illustrate how random slopes can be added to the regression model. Output 2.4 shows the output of the multilevel analysis on the example dataset in which not only a random intercept, but also a random slope is considered.

Output 2.4 looks slightly different from the earlier outputs that were shown. In the second line of Output 2.4 for instance, the regression coefficient for

Output 2.4. Results of a linear multilevel analysis of the relationship between total cholesterol and age, with both a random intercept and a random slope for age at the medical doctor level

```
total cholesterol_ij ~ N(XB, Ω)
total cholesterol_ij = β_0ij cons + β_1j age_ij
β_0ij = 2,8800(0,4009) + u_0j + e_0ij
β_1j = 0,0501(0,0058) + u_1j

|u_0j|  ~ N(0, Ω_u) : Ω_u = [1,4426(0,7780)                        ]
|u_1j|                      [-0,0172(0,0106)  0,0003(0,0002)]

[e_0ij] ~ N(0, Ω_e) : Ω_e = [0,3137(0,0217)]

-2*loglikelihood(IGLS) = 799,9644(441 of 441 cases in use)
```

age is indicated by β_{1j}. The subscript j indicates that the regression coefficients are allowed to differ between the medical doctors (remember that the subscript j stands for medical doctor). In the fourth line of the output it can be seen that this β_{1j} consists of the regression coefficient that we are interested in, and a variance parameter (u_{1j}), which is the variance of the regression coefficients for age for the different medical doctors. The magnitude of this variance (and the corresponding standard error) is shown in the variance matrix in the fifth and sixth line of the output. The first value of the matrix (i.e. 1.4426) reflects the variance of the intercepts, while the last value of the matrix (i.e. 0.0003) reflects the variance of the slopes. There is also another value shown in the matrix (i.e. −0.0172). This is the covariance between the random intercept and the random slope, which is also known as the correlation between the random intercept and the random slope or the interaction between the random intercept and the random slope. For the interpretation of this covariance, the sign is probably the most important. In the example there is a negative sign, which indicates an inverse relationship between the random intercept and the random slope. In other words, for medical doctors with a relatively high intercept, a relatively low slope is observed (see Figure 2.8). On the other hand, a positive sign of the covariance between a random intercept and a random slope indicates that the group with a relatively high intercept also has a relatively high slope.

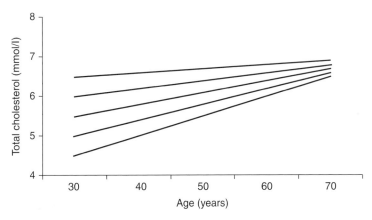

Figure 2.8. Illustration of a situation with a negative covariance between a random intercept and a random slope; patients with a relatively high intercept have a relatively low slope.

To evaluate the necessity of adding a random slope to the model, again the likelihood ratio test can be used. To do so, the -2 log likelihood of the model with only a random intercept (809.3788; from Output 2.3) has to be compared to the -2 log likelihood of the model with both a random intercept and a random slope (799.9644; from Output 2.4). The difference between the two is 9.4144, which follows a Chi-square distribution with two degrees of freedom. Two degrees of freedom, because not only the variance of the slopes has to be estimated, but also the covariance between the random intercept and the random slope. The latter is not really required, but it is a natural consequence of estimating two random variances. Evaluating 9.4144 on a Chi-square distribution with two degrees of freedom gives a p-value of less than 0.001. So, it is not only necessary to correct for medical doctor (i.e. to have a random intercept), but it is also necessary to have an interaction between age and medical doctor in the model (i.e. to have a random slope). The most important information, however, is shown in the fourth line of the output. The regression coefficient for age is 0.0501, with a standard error of 0.0058. The corresponding Wald statistic is $(0.0501/0.0058)^2 = 74.6$ (which is again highly significant) and the corresponding 95% CI ranges from 0.0387 to 0.0615.

One thing that is rather surprising is the high variance for the intercepts, compared to the variance resulting from the analysis when only a random intercept was considered (i.e. 1.4426 compared to 0.3686). This high value has to do with the fact that the intercept in this example does not have a real interpretation. Total cholesterol values when age is zero are not really relevant when the age range is between 44 and 86 years. In a situation with only a random intercept this does not influence the variance between the intercepts, because the difference between the regression lines is equal at each age (see, for instance, Figure 2.3). However, when the slopes of the regression lines differ, this can have a major influence on the variance of the intercepts when the value of the intercept is non-informative.

A possible way in which to make the intercept more interpretable is to use the centred value of the independent variable in the analysis. In our example this can be done by subtracting the average age from all individual (patient) observations. The results of this subtraction is that the average age in the dataset will be zero, and therefore the intercept can be interpreted as the total cholesterol value for the average age. Output 2.5 shows the results of a multilevel analysis with both a random intercept and a random slope when age is centred. The regression coefficient (and random variance) for age is (of course) exactly the same as before, but the magnitude of the intercept and the variance of the intercept have changed considerably. It can further be seen that the variance of the intercept has more or less the same value as in the analysis with only a random intercept.

Output 2.5. Results of a linear multilevel analysis of the relationship between total cholesterol and age, with both a random intercept and a random slope for age at the medical doctor level, when age is centred

---

total cholesterol$_{ij}$ ~ N(XB, Ω)
total cholesterol$_{ij}$ = β_{0ij}cons + β_{1j}age centred$_{ij}$
β_{0ij} = 5,9712(0,1756) + u_{0j} + e_{0ij}
β_{1j} = 0,0501(0,0058) + u_{1j}

$\begin{bmatrix} u_{0j} \\ u_{1j} \end{bmatrix}$ ~ N(0, Ω_u) : Ω_u = $\begin{bmatrix} 0,3611(0,1511) \\ -0,0004(0,0035) & 0,0003(0,0002) \end{bmatrix}$

$[e_{0ij}]$ ~ N(0, Ω_e) : Ω_e = [0,3137(0,0217)]

-2*loglikelihood(IGLS) = 799,9634(441 of 441 cases in use)

2.6 Multilevel analysis with more than two levels

Up to now, only a relatively simple situation has been considered, in which the patient observations were clustered within the medical doctors. It is, however, also possible that the different medical doctors come from the same hospital or institution, and that the observations within the medical doctors are therefore clustered within institutions (see Figure 2.9).

It is not surprising that this clustering within a higher level can be treated in the same way as has been described for the clustering of the patient observations within the medical doctor. So, also for the different institutions the variance of the intercepts can be estimated, and the variances of the regression coefficients reflecting the relationship between total cholesterol and age (i.e. the slopes) can also be estimated.

2.6.1 Example

Output 2.6 shows the descriptives of the example dataset described in the earlier sections, but it also includes the institution variable.

From Output 2.6 it can be seen that the 12 medical doctors 'belong' to 6 institutions. All other variables were already explained in Section 2.1.

Output 2.7 shows the results of the multilevel analysis in which a random intercept is assumed for medical doctor as well as for institution.

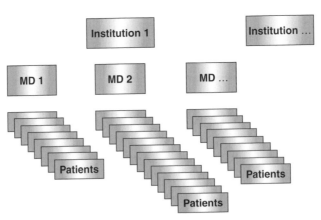

Figure 2.9. Three-level multilevel structure; patients are clustered within medical doctors and medical doctors are clustered within institutions.

Output 2.6. Descriptive information regarding the example dataset

5 institution		Refresh	Categories	Help
Name	**n**	**missing**	**min**	**max**
1 total cholesterol	441	0	3,9	8,86
2 medical doctor	441	0	1	12
3 age	441	0	44	86
4 id	441	0	1	441
5 institution	441	0	1	6
6 cons	441	0	1	1

Output 2.7. Results of a linear multilevel analysis of the relationship between total cholesterol and age with a random intercept at both the medical doctor level and the institution level

total cholesterol$_{ijk}$ ~ N(XB, Ω)

total cholesterol$_{ijk}$ = β_{0ijk}cons + 0,0494(0,0031)age$_{ijk}$

β_{0ijk} = 2,9162(0,3083) + v_{0k} + u_{0jk} + e_{0ijk}

$[v_{0k}]$ ~ N(0, Ω_v) : Ω_v = [0,3372(0,2067)]

$[u_{0jk}]$ ~ N(0, Ω_u) : Ω_u = [0,0315(0,0234)]

$[e_{0ijk}]$ ~ N(0, Ω_e) : Ω_e = [0,3315(0,0226)]

-2*loglikelihood(IGLS) = 799,8273(441 of 441 cases in use)

From the first line of Output 2.7 it can be seen that the outcome variable is measured on three levels. It was already known that subscript i stands for the lowest level, i.e. the patient, and that subscript j stands for the second level, i.e. the medical doctor. Subscript k is added to the outcome variable, which indicates that a third level is present, i.e. the institution. From the second and the third line of Output 2.7 it can be seen that (indeed) the intercept is considered to be random on all three levels. First of all, the β_0, has three subscripts, and after the intercept of 2.9162 and the corresponding standard error of 0.3083, three variances are added: the remaining unexplained variance (e_{0ijk}), the variance of the intercepts on the medical doctor level (u_{0jk}), and the variance of the intercepts on the institution level (v_{0k}). The magnitudes of the three variances are shown in the next three lines of the output. To evaluate the necessity of allowing a random intercept on the institution level, the results of this analysis must be compared to the results of the analysis with only a random intercept on the medical doctor level (see Output 2.3). This evaluation is made with the likelihood ratio test. The $-2\log$ likelihood of the model with only a random intercept on the medical doctor level was 809.3788, while the $-2\log$ likelihood of the model with both a random intercept on the medical doctor level and the institution level is 799.8273. The difference between the two is 9.5515, which is Chi-square distributed with one degree of freedom (only the random variance of the intercepts on the institution level is added to the model), which is highly significant. What can be seen is that the random variance of the intercepts on the medical doctor level is almost totally shifted to the random variance of the intercepts on the institution level. This means that almost all variance in intercepts observed between medical doctors is due to the variance in intercepts between institutions.

The next step in the analysis is to add random coefficients for the relationship with age to the regression model. At first, only a random slope for medical doctor is considered (Output 2.8).

Output 2.8. Results of a linear multilevel analysis of the relationship between total cholesterol and age with a random intercept at both the medical doctor level and the institution level and a random slope for age at the medical doctor level

---

```
total cholesterolᵢⱼₖ ~ N(XB, Ω)
```
$$\text{total cholesterol}_{ijk} \sim N(XB,\ \Omega)$$
$$\text{total cholesterol}_{ijk} = \beta_{0ijk}\text{cons} + \beta_{1j}\text{age}_{ijk}$$
$$\beta_{0ijk} = 2,8500\,(0,4132) + v_{0k} + u_{0jk} + e_{0ijk}$$
$$\beta_{1j} = 0,0505\,(0,0057) + u_{1jk}$$

$$[v_{0k}] \sim N(0,\ \Omega_v)\ :\ \Omega_v = [0,3437\,(0,2077)]$$

$$\begin{bmatrix} u_{0jk} \\ u_{1jk} \end{bmatrix} \sim N(0,\ \Omega_u)\ :\ \Omega_u = \begin{bmatrix} 0,8819(0,5589) & \\ -0,0149(0,0092) & 0,0003(0,0002) \end{bmatrix}$$

$$[e_{0ijk}] \sim N(0,\ \Omega_e)\ :\ \Omega_e = [0,3139\,(0,0217)]$$

$$-2*\text{loglikelihood(IGLS)} = 789,6476\ (441\ \text{of}\ 441\ \text{cases in use})$$

The fact that a random slope for medical doctor is considered can be seen from the regression coefficient for age, which has the subscript *j*. After the actual value of the regression coefficient for age (i.e. 0.0505) and corresponding standard error (i.e. 0.0057), an additional variance parameter (u_{1jk}) is added. That variance parameter stands for a random variance in the relationship between total cholesterol and age on the medical doctor level. The necessity of this variance can again be evaluated by comparing the -2 log likelihood of the model with this additional variance (789.6476) with the -2 log likelihood of the model without the additional variance (799.8273). The difference between the two (10.1797) follows a Chi-square distribution with two degrees of freedom (the variance of the slopes on the medical doctor level and the covariance between the intercepts and slopes on the medical doctor level), which is highly significant.

The last possibility for a random coefficient in the present model is allowing the regression coefficient with age to be random for each institution. Output 2.9 shows the results of the analysis in which the intercepts as well as the slopes were assumed to be random on both the medical doctor level and the institution level.

Output 2.9. Results of a linear multilevel analysis of the relationship between total cholesterol and age with a random intercept at both the medical doctor level and the institution level and a random slope for age at both the medical doctor level and the institution level

$$\text{total cholesterol}_{ijk} \sim N(XB, \; \Omega)$$

$$\text{total cholesterol}_{ijk} = \beta_{0ijk}\text{cons} + \beta_{1jk}\text{age}_{ijk}$$

$$\beta_{0ijk} = 2,8799(0,4009) + v_{0k} + u_{0jk} + e_{0ijk}$$

$$\beta_{1jk} = 0,0501(0,0058) + v_{1k} + u_{1jk}$$

$$\begin{bmatrix} v_{0k} \\ v_{1k} \end{bmatrix} \sim N(0, \; \Omega_v) : \Omega_v = \begin{bmatrix} 0,0000(0,0000) & \\ 0,0000(0,0000) & 0,0000(0,0000) \end{bmatrix}$$

$$\begin{bmatrix} u_{0jk} \\ u_{1jk} \end{bmatrix} \sim N(0, \; \Omega_u) : \Omega_u = \begin{bmatrix} 1,4428(0,7780) & \\ -0,0172(0,0106) & 0,0003(0,0002) \end{bmatrix}$$

$$[e_{0ijk}] \sim N(0, \; \Omega_e) : \Omega_e = [0,3137(0,0217)]$$

$$-2*\text{loglikelihood}(IGLS) = 799,9617(441 \text{ of } 441 \text{ cases in use})$$

A random slope on both the medical doctor and the institution level is indicated by the fact that the regression coefficient for age β_1 has the subscripts j and k, and that after the regression coefficient in the fourth line of Output 2.9, two additional variances are shown: one (u_{ijk}) for the variance of the regression coefficient for age on the medical doctor level, and one (v_{ik}) for the variance of the regression coefficient for age on the institution level. When the magnitude of the variances is considered, it can be seen that all variances on the institution level are zero, and although that is quite strange, this is often the case in models with a lot of random coefficients. The conclusion from all these zeros is that the last random coefficient (i.e. a random slope on the institution level) cannot be estimated accurately and therefore it can be considered as unimportant. So, the conclusion that can be drawn from all the analyses is that the most efficient way to estimate the relationship between total cholesterol and age is a model with random intercepts on both the medical doctor level and the institution level and a random slope on the medical doctor level. Therefore, the most appropriate estimate of the relationship between total cholesterol and age can be found in Output 2.8. The point estimate is 0.0505 and the corresponding standard error can be used to estimate the 95% CI around the point estimate. This 95% CI ranges from 0.0393 to 0.0617. The p-value of the (linear) relationship between total cholesterol and age can be derived from the Wald statistic, which is $(0.0505/0.0057)^2 = 78.5$. On a Chi-square distribution with one degree of freedom the corresponding p-value is <0.001.

2.7 Assumptions in multilevel analysis[1]

Because linear multilevel analysis is an extension of 'standard' linear regression analysis, all assumptions for 'standard' linear regression analysis also hold for multilevel analysis. So, the continuous outcome variable should be normally distributed; i.e. the residuals should be normally distributed. As in 'standard' linear regression analysis, this can be investigated by producing normal plots (see for details: Goldstein and Healy, 1995; Goldstein and

---

[1] For the way in which to check the assumptions in MLwiN, reference is made to the software manual (Rasbash et al., 2003) Chapters 3 and 15.

Spiegelhalter, 1996). Moreover, the residuals should be uncorrelated. In most multilevel studies this should not be a big problem, because the reason for performing a multilevel analysis in the first place, is that there are correlated observations (i.e. correlated residuals) in the data to be analysed. So, basically, by using multilevel analysis the problem of these correlated residuals is more or less solved. However, there are research situations in which the use of multilevel analysis only partly solves the problem of the correlated residuals. This is, for instance, often the case in longitudinal studies (see Section 6.6.1).

An additional assumption that is typical for multilevel analysis was already mentioned in the earlier sections, i.e. the random intercepts and the random slopes must be normally distributed. Whether or not this is a reasonable assumption can, for instance, be investigated by analysing the different groups (i.e. medical doctors) separately. It should be realised that this is not always possible (especially when many groups are involved).

In addition to checking the assumptions of the linear multilevel analysis, it can also be important to investigate whether the model coefficients are influenced by certain data-points or whether outliers are present in the analysed dataset. Because of the multilevel structure of the data, outliers (or influencing data points) can occur at different levels. Observations of patients can influence the overall relationship that is analysed, or can be outliers at patient level. On the other hand, a single patient observation can also be an outlier for the particular medical doctor to whom that patient 'belongs'; in other words, the patient observation can be an outlier at the medical doctor level. For detailed information regarding outliers and influencing data points in multilevel studies, reference is made to Atkinson (1986), Barnett and Lewis (1994), Lawrence (1995), or Langford and Lewis (1998).

2.8 Comments

2.8.1 Which regression coefficients can be assumed to be random?

From the analyses discussed in this chapter it can be seen that on the lowest level (i.e. the patient observations) only the intercept is considered to be random. This random intercept at patient level was the overall error variance of the regression analysis. Some people wonder why the other regression coefficients are not considered to be random at patient level. This is, however, not possible. In the example, the relationship between total cholesterol and age

was considered. For each patient this relationship is based on only one observation, and each patient has one age and one total cholesterol value. So, on at
patient level there are no slopes! Considering a random slope on at patient
level therefore makes no sense[2]. A general rule concerning random regression
coefficients is that they can only be considered to be random at a level above
that on which they are measured. In the situation in the present example this
means that because age is measured at patient level, it can only be assumed
to be random on the levels above the patient level (i.e. at the medical doctor
level and at the institution level). In line with this, if a variable was measured
at the medical doctor level (for instance gender or age of the medical doctor)
this variable can only be assumed to be random at the institution level.

2.8.2 Random regression coefficients versus fixed regression coefficients

Within multilevel analysis, a distinction must be made between fixed and
random regression coefficients. It should be realised that this distinction differs from the distinction between random and fixed factors in the traditional analysis of variance. In analysis of variance, a random factor is defined
as 'a categorical variable in which the groups are a random sample of all possible groups about which conclusions are desired' (e.g. medical doctor or
institution), while a fixed factor is defined as 'a categorical variable about
which conclusions are desired for every group' (e.g. gender). In multilevel
analysis, however, a fixed regression coefficient is just the regression coefficient itself. In principle, all regression coefficients of a multilevel analysis are
fixed, because in general one is interested in the magnitude of the regression
coefficients. In addition to the fixed part of the regression coefficient, each
regression coefficient can also be considered to be random (depending on
the level on which the variable is measured (see Section 2.8.1)). This random part of the regression coefficient is the variation of the regression coefficient between the groups considered (e.g. medical doctors, school classes,
etc.). The term random is probably not the most appropriate in this respect,
because the regression coefficients are not really 'random'; they are assumed
to be different for different groups.

---

[2] It should be realised that in the MLwiN software it is possible to add a random slope at the
lowest level, although it makes no sense.

2.8.3 Maximum likelihood versus restricted maximum likelihood

In all the outputs presented so far, IGLS was printed between brackets after the $-2\log$ likelihoods of the model. IGLS stands for Iterative Generalised Least Squares (in fact it is rather strange that the estimation procedure is called IGLS, because the regression coefficients and variances are estimated by maximum likelihood (ML)). There is also another procedure that can be used to estimate the regression coefficients and variances, i.e. Restricted Maximum Likelihood (REML). In the MLwiN software this technique is known as Restricted Iterative Generalised Least Squares (RIGLS). It should be noted that in some software packages, such as SAS and SPSS, the REML estimation procedure is the default (see also Chapter 9). There is no real consensus concerning the 'best' estimation procedure. It is often argued that REML is 'better' for the estimation of random variances, while ML is 'better' for the estimation of the (fixed) regression coefficients. In general, the (fixed) regression coefficients are of major interest, so, therefore, in the examples presented in this book ML estimation procedure will be used. To illustrate the differences between the ML and the REML estimation procedures, the relationship between age (centred) and total cholesterol with both a random intercept and a random slope on the medical doctor level (results shown in Output 2.5) was also estimated with REML. The results of both analyses are shown in Table 2.1.

From Table 2.1 it can be seen that the differences between the two estimation procedures are only marginal. Not surprisingly, the only (small) differences were observed for the variance of the random intercept and the $-2\log$ likelihood.

Table 2.1. Relationship between age (centred) and total cholesterol, estimated with ML estimation procedure and with a REML procedure

	ML estimate	REML estimate
Intercept	5.97 (0.18)	5.97 (0.18)
Age	0.050 (0.006)	0.050 (0.006)
Random intercept at the medical doctor level	0.36 (0.15)	0.39 (0.16)
Random slope for age at the medical doctor level	0.0003 (0.0002)	0.0003 (0.0002)
$-2\log$ likelihood	799.9634	800.0581

3

What do we gain by applying multilevel analysis?

3.1 Introduction

Before multilevel analysis was developed, the problem of correlated observations within, for instance, medical doctors was tackled in two ways: either ignoring the fact that the observations are correlated or combining the correlated observations into one value. In fact, both methods are still frequently used. Ignoring the fact that the observations are correlated indicates that all observations are analysed as independent. In Chapter 2, this method was called 'naive' analysis, the advantage of which is that 'standard' regression analysis can be used. This way of analysing clustered data is also referred to as the 'disaggregation' method. The other possibility is not to ignore the dependency of the observations, but to analyse the group observations (i.e. made by each medical doctor) instead of the individual observations. Therefore, some sort of average value of the observations for each group must first be calculated and then these averages can be used as outcome in a 'standard' regression analysis. This method is referred to as the 'aggregation' method. To answer the question: 'What do we gain by using multilevel analysis?', it is interesting to compare the results obtained from these three types of analysis: the 'naive/disaggregation' method, the 'aggregation' method, and the (more sophisticated) multilevel analysis.

3.2 Example with a balanced dataset

In this example we use a dataset from a randomised controlled trial. The outcome variable in this experimental study is a certain continuous health outcome. The total study population consists of 200 patients, randomly divided into an intervention group and a control group. The intervention was performed by 20 medical doctors, and in this balanced dataset each medical doctor had 10 patients. The randomisation was performed on the patients, which means that for each medical doctor half of the patients were allocated to the intervention group, and the other half to the control group. Output 3.1 shows the dataset that is used in this example.

Output 3.1. Descriptive information regarding the balanced dataset used in the example

1 health outcome			Refresh	Categories	Help

Name	n	missing	min	max	
1 health outcome	200	0	4,9	8,92	
2 medical doctor	200	0	1	20	
3 id	200	0	1	200	
4 intervention	200	0	0	1	
5 cons	200	0	1	1	

The first analysis that was performed was a 'naive/disaggregated' analysis, or, in other words, all patients are considered to be independent. Output 3.2 shows the output of this analysis in MLwiN. The results are (of course) exactly the same as the results obtained from a 'standard' linear regression analysis. To illustrate this, Output 3.3 shows the output of this 'naive/disaggregated' analysis performed in SPSS. The only difference is that in 'standard' linear regression analysis performed in SPSS the regression coefficients are estimated with ordinary least squares, while with multilevel analysis the regression coefficients are estimated with maximum likelihood. As a consequence of this difference, in 'standard' linear regression analysis a t-statistic and a t-distribution are used to evaluate whether or not the effect of the intervention is significant. With multilevel analysis (in MLwiN), on the other hand, this is done with the Wald statistic and the Chi-square distribution (see Section 2.2). The magnitude of the regression coefficient and the standard error will (of course) be the same for both methods, and when there is a large study population the corresponding p-values will also be the same.

Output 3.2. Results of a 'naive/disaggregated' analysis performed in MLwiN on a balanced dataset to determine the effects of the intervention on a certain health outcome

```
health outcome_ij ~ N(XB, Ω)
heath outcome_ij = β_0icons + 0,289(0,121)intervention_ij
β_0i = 6,501(0,085) + e_0ij

[e_0ij] ~ N(0, Ω_e) : Ω_e = [0,727(0,073)]

-2*loglikelihood(IGLS) = 503,699(200 of 200 cases in use)
```

Output 3.3. Results of a 'naive/disaggregated' analysis performed in SPSS on a balanced dataset to determine the effects of the intervention on a certain health outcome

Coefficients[a]

Model		Unstandardized Coefficients		t	Sig.
		B	Std. Error		
1	(Constant)	6,501	,086	75,888	,000
	intervention	,289	,121	2,387	,018

[a]Dependent variable: health outcome.

From Outputs 3.2 and 3.3 it can be seen that the intervention effect was 0.289, with a standard error of 0.121. Based on the multilevel analysis, the 95% confidence interval (CI) of this intervention effect is $0.289 \pm 1.96 \times 0.121 = [0.052–0.526]$. Output 3.4 shows the results of the multilevel analysis, not ignoring the dependency of the observations. In the multilevel analysis, both a random intercept and a random regression coefficient for the intervention variable (a random slope) were allowed.

When a multilevel analysis is performed with random regression coefficients, the intervention effect remains exactly the same (i.e. 0.289), but the standard error increases from 0.121 to 0.175 (see Outputs 3.2 and 3.4). The 95% CI around this intervention effect is therefore $0.289 \pm 1.96 \times 0.175 =$

Output 3.4. Results of a multilevel analysis on a balanced dataset to determine the effects of the intervention on a certain health outcome. Both a random intercept and a random slope for the intervention variable are assumed

```
health outcomeᵢⱼ ~ N(XB, Ω)
health outcomeᵢⱼ = β₀ᵢⱼcons + β₁ⱼinterventionᵢⱼ
β₀ᵢⱼ = 6,501(0,110) + u₀ⱼ + e₀ᵢⱼ
β₁ⱼ = 0,289(0,175) + u₁ⱼ
```

$$\begin{bmatrix} u_{0j} \\ u_{1j} \end{bmatrix} \sim N(0, \; \Omega_u) \; : \; \Omega_u = \begin{bmatrix} 0{,}162(0{,}078) & \\ -0{,}071(0{,}094) & 0{,}449(0{,}195) \end{bmatrix}$$

$$[e_{0ij}] \sim N(0, \; \Omega_e) \; : \; \Omega_e = [0{,}412(0{,}046)]$$

```
-2*loglikelihood(IGLS) = 448,579(200 of 200 cases in use)
```

[−0.054–0.632], which is no longer significant. The fact that the standard error obtained from the multilevel analysis is higher than the standard error obtained from the 'naive/disaggregated' analysis is not surprising. In the analysis that ignores the dependency of the observations, each observation is considered to provide 100% new information. In a multilevel analysis, a correction is made for medical doctor, which means that the information provided by a patient 'belonging' to the same medical doctor does not give 100% new information, but less. The magnitude of the new information provided by each individual patient depends on the magnitude of the intra-class correlation coefficient (ICC). The higher the ICC, the less new information provided by a patient 'belonging' to the same medical doctor, and the higher the standard error of the multilevel analysis, compared to the 'naive/disaggregated' analysis.

When the analysis is performed on the average health outcomes of the patients of the 20 medical doctors, it can be seen that the regression coefficient of this 'aggregated' analysis is exactly the same as for the other two analyses. However, because only 40 observations are analysed (i.e. the average values of the 20 medical doctors for the intervention and control group), the standard error of the regression coefficient is much higher than in the other two analyses (see Output 3.5).

Output 3.5. Results of an 'aggregated' analysis on a balanced dataset performed in SPSS to determine the effects of the intervention on a certain health outcome

Coefficients[a]

Model		Unstandardized Coefficients		t	Sig.
		B	Std. Error		
1	(Constant)	6,501	,145	44,966	,000
	intervention	,289	,204	1,414	,165

[a] Dependent variable: average health outcome.

3.3 Example with an unbalanced dataset

The differences between a 'naive/disaggregated' analysis, a multilevel analysis, and an 'aggregated' analysis are different when the dataset is unbalanced. In the following example, the dataset used in the example in Section 3.2 is changed in such a way that for half of the medical doctors, only six patients (equally divided into intervention and control groups) are included in the study. So, instead of 200 patients in the earlier example, this dataset includes 160 patients. Output 3.6 shows the results of the analysis ignoring the dependency of the observations within the medical doctors (i.e. the results of the 'naive/disaggregated' analysis).

Output 3.6. Results of a 'naive/disaggregated' analysis performed in MLwiN on an unbalanced dataset to determine the effects of the intervention on a certain health outcome

$$\text{health outcome}_{ij} \sim N(XB, \ \Omega)$$
$$\text{heath outcome}_{ij} = \beta_{0i}\text{cons} + 0,271(0,136)\text{intervention}_{ij}$$
$$\beta_{0i} = 6,582(0,096) + e_{0ij}$$
$$[e_{0ij}] \sim N(0, \ \Omega_e) \ : \ \Omega_e = [0,740(0,083)]$$
$$-2*\text{loglikelihood}(IGLS) = 405,792(160 \text{ of } 160 \text{ cases in use})$$

From Output 3.6 it can be seen that the intervention effect is 0.271, with a standard error of 0.136. This results in a 95% CI, ranging from 0.004 to 0.540. The corresponding p-value, which can be derived from the Wald test $[(0.271/0.136)^2 = 3.97]$, is 0.046. When a multilevel analysis is performed (again with both a random intercept and a random slope for the intervention variable), not only the standard error of the intervention effect changes, but also the intervention effect itself (see Output 3.7). The intervention effect is now 0.187, with a 95% CI ranging from -0.23 to 0.61, and the p-value for this intervention effect is no longer significant, i.e. 0.383; derived from the Wald statistic $([0.187/0.215]^2 = 0.76)$.

Output 3.7. Results of a multilevel analysis on an unbalanced dataset to determine the effects of the intervention on a certain health outcome. Both a random intercept and a random slope for the intervention variable are assumed

```
health outcome_{ij} ~ N(XB, Ω)
health outcome_{ij} = β_{0ij}cons + β_{1j}intervention_{ij}
β_{0ij} = 6,559(0,116) + u_{0j} + e_{0ij}
β_{1j} = 0,187(0,215) + u_{1j}

|u_{0j}|              | 0,167(0,086)               |
|u_{1j}| ~ N(0, Ω_u) : Ω_u = |-0,153(0,126)  0,714(0,292)|

[e_{0ij}] ~ N(0, Ω_e) : Ω_e = [0,397(0,051)]

-2*loglikelihood(IGLS) = 363,628(160 of 160 cases in use)
```

When an 'aggregated' analysis is applied to this unbalanced dataset, both the intervention effect and the corresponding standard error are different from the results of the previous analyses (see Output 3.8).

3.4 Cluster randomisation

The examples described in Sections 3.2 and 3.3 are related to a randomisation at patient level. This means that in the multilevel analysis the intervention effect can also be considered random among medical doctors, i.e. it was

Output 3.8. Results of an 'aggregated' analysis on an unbalanced dataset performed in SPSS to determine the effects of the intervention on a certain health outcome

```
Coefficientsᵃ
```

Model		Unstandardized coefficients		t	Sig.
		B	Std. Error		
1	(Constant)	6,546	,160	40,894	,000
	intervention	,181	,226	,799	,429

```
ᵃDependent variable: average health outcome.
```

possible to assume a random slope for the intervention variable. When a cluster randomisation design is used, i.e. when the randomisation is not carried out at patient level, but at the medical doctor level, the intervention effect can not be considered to be random among the medical doctors (remember the rule that random regression coefficients can only be considered at a level above the level on which the specific variable is measured).

Table 3.1. Results of a 'naive/disaggregated' analysis, a multilevel analysis, and an 'aggregated' analysis on a dataset in which a cluster randomisation is performed, i.e. the randomisation is carried out at the medical doctor level

	Intervention effect	Standard error	p-value
Balanced dataset[1]			
'Naive/disaggregation'	0.259	0.121	0.032
Multilevel analysis	0.259	0.213	0.224
'Aggregation'	0.259	0.225	0.265
Unbalanced dataset[2]			
'Naive/disaggregation'	0.176	0.137	0.199
Multilevel analysis	0.126	0.218	0.563
'Aggregation'	0.087	0.228	0.707

[1] In the balanced dataset 200 patients were included, equally divided among the 20 medical doctors.
[2] In the unbalanced dataset, for half of the medical doctors only six patients were included, resulting in a total of 160 patients.

However, the differences and equalities between a 'naive/disaggregated' analysis, a multilevel analysis, and an 'aggregated' analysis are comparable to the differences described for a dataset in which the randomisation is carried out at patient level. Table 3.1 summarises the results of the three different types of analyses on the dataset with a cluster randomisation.

3.5 Conclusion

Irrespective of the way in which randomisation is performed (i.e. either at patient level or on the medical doctor level), the differences between a 'naive/disaggregated' analysis, a multilevel analysis and an 'aggregated' analysis depend on whether or not the dataset is balanced. If the dataset is balanced, the only difference between the methods is observed in the standard error of the regression coefficients. However, when the dataset is unbalanced, there is a difference between the regression coefficients and the corresponding standard errors in the three methods.

For more detailed (mathematical) information related to the topic addressed in this chapter, reference is made, for instance, to Neuhaus and Kalbfleisch, 1998; Opdenakker and van Damme, 2000; Wampold and Serlin, 2000; Hutchinson and Healy, 2001; Tranmer and Steel, 2001; Moerbeek et al., 2003a or Moerbeek, 2004.

4

Multilevel analysis with different outcome variables

4.1 Introduction

In the foregoing chapters, multilevel analysis was explained with examples from studies with continuous outcome variables (i.e. linear multilevel analysis). One of the biggest advantages of multilevel analysis is that it can be used for the analysis of other kinds of outcome variables as well. Logistic multilevel analysis can be used for dichotomous outcome variables, multinomial logistic multilevel analysis can be used for categorical outcome variables, and Poisson multilevel analysis can be used for so-called 'count' outcome variables. Furthermore, it is possible to perform a multilevel survival analysis, although the necessary software has not yet been fully developed for this type of analysis.

4.2 Logistic multilevel analysis

The general principles behind logistic multilevel analysis (i.e. multilevel analysis with a dichotomous outcome variable) are the same as those described in Chapter 2 for linear multilevel analysis. So, in general, multilevel analysis with a dichotomous outcome variable is a logistic regression analysis in which an additional correction can be made for categorical variables, such as medical doctor or school. It should be realised that the estimation of the random variances, in particular, is mathematically quite difficult, and that different software packages use different estimation procedures. Unfortunately, however, these different procedures often lead to different results (see Chapter 9 for further information about the use of the various software packages).

The use of logistic multilevel analysis can best be illustrated by analysing an example dataset. As in the earlier chapters, the dataset will be analysed in MLwiN, and it is the same dataset that was used in the example with continuous outcome variables; the only difference is that now total cholesterol is not related to age, but the outcome is hypercholesterolemia (yes versus no). Output 4.1 shows descriptive information regarding the dataset used in the example.

Output 4.1. Descriptive information regarding the dataset used in the example to explain logistic multilevel analysis

	Name	n	missing	min	max	
	1 hypercholestei		**Refresh**	**Categories**	**❓ Help**	
1	hypercholesterolemia	441	0	0	1	
2	medical doctor	441	0	1	12	
3	age	441	0	44	86	
4	id	441	0	1	441	
5	cons	441	0	1	1	
6	bcons	441	0	1	1	
7	denom	441	0	1	1	

As can be seen from Output 4.1, again there are 441 observations, 12 medical doctors, and a patient age-range between 44 and 86 years. It cannot be seen from Output 4.1, but the prevalence of hypercholesterolemia in the example dataset is 39%. The column *cons* was already seen in the chapters dealing with continuous outcome variables, and was necessary to estimate the intercept of the multilevel regression model (see Section 2.2). To perform a logistic multilevel analysis in MLwiN software, in addition to the column *cons*, two additional columns of ones are needed. The column *bcons* is needed to define the error variance of the logistic regression model, but this will be explained later. The column *denom* is a feature of the MLwiN software that is comparable, for instance, to the *weight cases* option in SPSS. This feature makes it possible to use a so-called 'grouped' data structure, which can be, especially suitable when the dataset consists only of dichotomous variables. In the dataset in Table 4.1, for instance, there are only eight

Table 4.1. Illustration of a 'grouped' data structure with one dichotomous outcome and two dichotomous determinants

Outcome	Determinant 1	Determinant 2	Denom
0	0	0	20
0	0	1	10
0	1	0	5
0	1	1	10
1	0	0	20
1	0	1	25
1	1	0	40
1	1	1	20

combinations possible, and therefore there are only eight rows in the dataset. These eight rows represent 150 patients, 20 of whom, for instance, have 0 for the outcome variable and also 0 for the two determinants, while 10 of whom have 0 for the outcome variable and the first determinant, but 1 for the second determinant, etc. In most situations, however, each patient is presented in the dataset by a separate row, and then the variable *denom* is a row of ones.

Output 4.2 shows the results of a 'naive' logistic regression analysis of the relationship between hypercholesterolemia and age. In this first analysis all observations are assumed to be independent, i.e. no correction is made for medical doctor.

Output 4.2. Results of a 'naive' logistic multilevel analysis of the relationship between hypercholesterolemia and age

$$\left. \begin{array}{l} \text{hypercholesterolemia}_{ij} \sim \text{Binomial}(\text{denom}_{ij}, \pi_{ij}) \\ \text{hypercholesterolemia}_{ij} = \pi_{ij} + e_{0ij}\text{bcons}^* \end{array} \right|$$

$$\text{logit}(\pi_{ij}) = -6,825(0,819)\text{cons} + 0,102(0,013)\text{age}_{ij}$$

$$\text{bcons}^* = \text{bcons}[\pi_{ij}(1 - \pi_{ij})/\text{denom}_{ij}]^{0.5}$$

$$[e_{0ij}] \sim (0, \Omega_e) : \Omega_e = [1,000(0,000)]$$

The first line of Output 4.2 shows that we are dealing with a dichotomous outcome variable (i.e. a binomial distribution). In the second line of the output it can be seen that the dichotomous outcome variable hypercholesterolemia is modelled by the probability (π) and a certain 'error'. This looks a bit strange, but it is typical for logistic regression analysis. The 'error' (or 'residual') is already reflected in the probability, and therefore the *bcons* parameter (a row of ones) is needed. Again, it is a bit strange that this must explicitly be included in the model, because it is directly related to the fact that a logistic regression analysis is performed (therefore, in any other software package the addition of *bcons* is not necessary, because it is added automatically)[1]. The third line of the output shows the logistic regression model. The outcome variable is the 'logit of the probability' or, in other words, the natural log of the odds of having hypercholesterolemia. Again, this is exactly the same as in a 'standard' logistic regression analysis. From the output it can be seen that the regression coefficient for age = 0.102. This regression coefficient can be transformed into an odds ratio by taking EXP[regression coefficient]. In the example the odds ratio for age is therefore EXP[0.102] = 1.11. This means that for a difference of 1 year in age, the odds for hypercholesterolemia for the older patient is 1.11 times higher compared to the odds for hypercholesterolemia for the younger patient. In the same way the 95% confidence interval (CI) can be estimated: EXP[regression coefficient $\pm$ 1.96 times the standard error]. In the present example the 95% CI around the odds ratio of 1.11 ranges between 1.08 and 1.14. This is a relatively small odds ratio, with a narrow interval, which is due to the fact that it reflects the odds ratio related to only 1 year difference in age. From the 95% CI around the odds ratio, it can be seen that the corresponding odds ratio differs significantly from 1 (i.e. the value of 1, which reflects no relationship, does not lie within the interval). Comparable to the linear multilevel analysis (see Chapter 2), the actual *p*-value of the regression coefficient (i.e. the actual *p*-value of the odds ratio) can be derived from the Wald test. Again, the Wald statistic is defined by the regression coefficient divided by its standard error, and this magnitude squared follows a Chi-square distribution with one degree

---

[1] To perform a logistic multilevel analysis in MLwiN software, the variable *bcons* must be only random at the lowest level (not fixed), while the variable *cons* must not be random at the lowest level (fixed, and if necessary random on the levels other than the lowest level). However, in the 'new' version of MLwiN (i.e. Version 2.0) this is done automatically, and *bcons* is not needed anymore.

of freedom. In the example the Wald statistic is: $(0.102/0.013)^2 = 61.6$; which is highly significant ($p < 0.001$).

The last two lines of the output are related to the fact that a logistic regression analysis is performed, and will not be discussed in detail. What is important, however, is the fact that no $-2 \log$ likelihood is shown. This is because the parameters of the logistic multilevel analysis are estimated with quasi-likelihood instead of maximum likelihood (or restricted maximum likelihood), and therefore the $-2 \log$ likelihood can not be estimated.

Output 4.3 shows the result of a logistic multilevel analysis, in which a correction is made for medical doctor, or, in other words, a logistic regression analysis in which the intercept is allowed to vary among medical doctors.

Output 4.3. Results of a logistic multilevel analysis with a random intercept to determine the relationship between hypercholesterolemia and age

$$\left. \begin{array}{l} \text{hypercholesterolemia}_{ij} \sim \text{Binomial}(\text{denom}_{ij}, \ \pi_{ij}) \\ \text{hypercholesterolemia}_{ij} = \pi_{ij} + e_{0ij}\text{bcons}^* \end{array} \right|$$

$$\text{logit}(\pi_{ij}) = \beta_{1j}\text{cons} + 0,180(0,023)\text{age}_{ij}$$

$$\beta_{1j} = -12,051(1,680) + u_{1j}$$

$$[u_{1j}] \sim N(0, \ \Omega_u) : \Omega_u = [5,590(2,448)]$$

$$\text{bcons}^* = \text{bcons}[\pi_{ij}(1 - \pi_{ij})/\text{denom}_{ij}]^{0.5}$$

$$[e_{0ij}] \sim (0, \ \Omega_e) : \Omega_e = [1,000(0,000)]$$

The fact that a correction is made for medical doctor can be seen in the fourth line of Output 4.3. This line shows the intercept of the regression model, and the variance of that intercept (reflected by u_{1j}). The magnitude (i.e. 5.590) and the standard error (i.e. 2.448) of this variance are shown in the next line of the output. The question then arises is whether or not it is necessary to allow the intercepts to be different for the medical doctors; or, in other words; whether or not it is necessary to correct for medical doctor in this analysis. As there is no $-2 \log$ likelihood available, the likelihood ratio test can not be performed in this situation, so we need something else. One of the possibilities (and maybe the only one) is to use the magnitude of the variance in combination with the standard error of the variance. It is theoretically not correct to perform the Wald test on variance parameters, but it gives an indication of whether or not the variance of the intercepts is 'important'. In the present example the magnitude of the variance is 2.28 times higher than the corresponding standard error. It is difficult to provide cut-off values for this 'incorrect' test, but when the variance is more than 2 times higher than its own standard error, the variance 'must' be considered as important, and therefore the corresponding regression coefficient 'must' be allowed to be random. In this example, the variance of the intercept was 2.28 times higher than the standard error, so a random variance of the intercept 'must' be added to the logistic regression model.

Looking at the relationship between age and hypercholesterolemia, it can be seen that both the regression coefficient and the standard error have increased, compared to the results of the 'naive' analysis which were reported in Output 4.2. The fact that the standard error increases when a correction is made for medical doctor was already seen in the examples in the earlier chapters. This has to do with the fact that an individual patient 'belonging' to the same medical doctor does not provide 100% new information, while in the 'naive' analysis it is assumed that the observations of each patient are independent, and therefore all observations provide 100% new information. In fact, the differences between a 'naive' analysis, a multilevel analysis, and an 'aggregated' analysis for dichotomous outcomes are the same as those described in Chapter 3 for continuous outcomes. The odds ratio (and 95% CI) for age in the analysis correcting for medical doctor is 1.20 [1.14–1.25]. The Wald test again reveals a highly significant p-value ($p < 0.001$).

The next question that can be asked is whether or not it is necessary to allow the relationship between age and hypercholesterolemia to be different for the medical doctors. Or, in other words, is it necessary to allow a random slope for age? Output 4.4 shows the results of the analysis in which, in addition to a random intercept, a random slope with age is also considered.

From Output 4.4 it can be seen that both regression coefficients in the model (i.e. the intercept and the regression coefficient for age) are considered to be random. Both have a variance parameter (u_{1j} and u_{2j}, respectively) added to the actual regression coefficient. The fifth and sixth lines of the output show the magnitude of the different variances, as well as the value of

Output 4.4. Results of a logistic multilevel analysis with a random intercept and a random slope for age to determine the relationship between hypercholesterolemia and age

$$\left. \begin{aligned} \text{hypercholesterolemia}_{ij} &\sim \text{Binomial}(\text{denom}_{ij}, \pi_{ij}) \\ \text{hypercholesterolemia}_{ij} &= \pi_{ij} + e_{0ij}\text{bcons}^* \end{aligned} \right|$$

$$\text{logit}(\pi_{ij}) = \beta_{1j}\text{cons} + \beta_{2j}\text{age}_{ij}$$

$$\beta_{1j} = -12,063\,(1,685) + u_{1j}$$

$$\beta_{2j} = 0,180\,(0,024) + u_{2j}$$

$$\begin{bmatrix} u_{1j} \\ u_{2j} \end{bmatrix} \sim N(0, \Omega_u) : \Omega_u = \begin{bmatrix} 5,605(2,471) \\ 0,000(0,000) & 0,000(0,000) \end{bmatrix}$$

$$\text{bcons}^* = \text{bcons}\,[\pi_{ij}(1 - \pi_{ij})/\text{denom}_{ij}]^{0.5}$$

$$[e_{0ij}] \sim (0, \Omega_e) : \Omega_e = [1,000\,(0,000)]$$

the covariance (correlation or interaction) between the random intercept and the random slope for age. It can be seen that both the slope variance and the covariance are zero, which implies that in this particular situation a random slope for age can not be properly estimated and is, therefore, not necessary. So, in conclusion, the most appropriate way (i.e. model) to estimate the relationship between age and hypercholesterolemia is shown in Output 4.3, i.e. only allowing a random intercept.

It was already mentioned that it is rather difficult to estimate (in particular) the random variances in a logistic multilevel analysis. Therefore, many different estimation procedures exist (see Chapter 9 for details). Within the quasi-likelihood estimations in MLwiN, different estimation procedures are also available. In the examples, a so-called second order penalised quasi-likelihood (second order PQL) estimation procedure is used. Although there are still some ongoing discussions, a second order PQL estimation procedure is thought to be the most appropriate method (Nelder and Lee, 1992; Rodriguez and Goldman, 1995; Goldstein and Rasbash, 1996; Neuhaus and Lesparance, 1996; Greenland, 1997; Rodriguez and Goldman, 1997; Engel, 1998; Rodriguez and Goldman, 2001; Moerbeek et al., 2003b). The default estimation procedure is, however, a first order maximised quasi-likelihood (first order MQL) estimation procedure. To illustrate the difference between the estimation procedures, Outputs 4.5 (a logistic multilevel analysis with only a random intercept) and 4.6 (a logistic multilevel analysis with both a random intercept and a random slope for age) show the results of logistic multilevel analysis performed with a first order MQL estimation procedure.

Output 4.5. Results of a logistic multilevel analysis with a random intercept to determine the relationship between hypercholesterolemia and age estimated with a first order MQL estimation procedure

---

$$\text{hypercholesterolemia}_{ij} \sim \text{Binomial}(\text{denom}_{ij}, \pi_{ij})$$
$$\text{hypercholesterolemia}_{ij} = \pi_{ij} + e_{0ij}\text{bcons}^*$$

$$\text{logit}(\pi_{ij}) = \beta_{1j}\text{cons} + 0,102(0,013)\text{age}_{ij}$$

$$\beta_{1j} = -6,861(0,930) + u_{1j}$$

$$[u_{1j}] \sim N(0, \Omega_u): \Omega_u = [1,770(0,779)]$$

$$\text{bcons}^* = \text{bcons}[\pi_{ij}(1 - \pi_{ij})/\text{denom}_{ij}]^{0.5}$$

$$[e_{0ij}] \sim (0, \Omega_e): \Omega_e = [1,000(0,000)]$$

Output 4.6. Results of a logistic multilevel analysis with a random intercept and a random slope for age to determine the relationship between hypercholesterolemia and age estimated with a first order MQL estimation procedure

---

$$\text{hypercholesterolemia}_{ij} \sim \text{Binomial}(\text{denom}_{ij}, \pi_{ij})$$
$$\text{hypercholesterolemia}_{ij} = \pi_{ij} + e_{0ij}\text{bcons}^*$$

$$\text{logit}(\pi_{ij}) = \beta_{1j}\text{cons} + \beta_{2j}\text{age}_{ij}$$

$$\beta_{1j} = -6,740(1,539) + u_{1j}$$

$$\beta_{2j} = 0,100(0,022) + u_{2j}$$

$$\begin{bmatrix} u_{1j} \\ u_{2j} \end{bmatrix} \sim N(0, \Omega_u): \Omega_u = \begin{bmatrix} 19,176(11,481) & \\ -0,256(0,164) & 0,004(0,002) \end{bmatrix}$$

$$\text{bcons}^* = \text{bcons}[\pi_{ij}(1 - \pi_{ij})/\text{denom}_{ij}]^{0.5}$$

$$[e_{0ij}] \sim (0, \Omega_e): \Omega_e = [1,000(0,000)]$$

Surprisingly (or maybe not) the results are totally different. In the model with only a random intercept (Output 4.5), the regression coefficient for age is exactly the same as in the 'naive' analysis (Output 4.2). This also applies to the magnitude of the standard error. When a random slope for age is added to the model, and the parameters are estimated with a first order MQL estimation procedure, a random slope for age seems to be quite reasonable (Output 4.6). Furthermore, the regression coefficient for age is much lower than when a second order PQL estimation procedure is applied (compare Output 4.4 with Output 4.6).

It should be noted that the differences between a first order MQL estimation procedure and a second order PQL estimation procedure are not always the same as those found in the present example. In fact, the differences between these two procedures are rather unpredictable.

4.2.1 Intraclass correlation coefficient in logistic multilevel analysis

For continuous outcome variables it was mentioned that the dependency of the observations on a certain level could be estimated by the intraclass correlation coefficient (ICC) (see Section 2.3). The ICC was estimated as the ratio of the between group variance and the total variance. Due to the total variance is not directly available in a logistic model, an alternative way of estimating the ICC is provided by Equation (4.1):

$$\text{ICC} = \frac{\sigma^2_{\text{between}}}{\sigma^2_{\text{between}} + \left(\dfrac{\pi^2}{3}\right)} \tag{4.1}$$

where $\sigma^2_{\text{between}}$ = between group variance.

We can use Output 4.3 to estimate the ICC in the present example:

$$\text{ICC} = \frac{5.59}{5.59 + \left(\dfrac{3.14^2}{3}\right)} = 0.63$$

Although it is possible to estimate the ICC in a logistic multilevel analysis, it is questionable whether this should be done, mainly because a correlation coefficient for a dichotomous variable is very difficult to interpret. It is, therefore also suggested that a so-called 'median odds ratio' can be used as an alternative

ICC (Larsen et al., 2000; Larsen and Merlo, 2005). The theory behind the 'median odds ratio' sounds reasonable, but in practice it is not widely used.

For a more detailed mathematical explanation of logistic multilevel analysis, reference is made, for instance, to Mealli and Rampichini (1999), Omar and Thompson (2000), Carlin et al. (2001), Turner et al. (2001), and Goldstein (2003).

4.3 Multinomial logistic multilevel analysis

When the outcome variable is categorical, multinomial logistic multilevel analysis can be applied. As for all other multilevel analysis, multinomial logistic multilevel analysis is an extension of 'standard' multinomial logistic regression analysis. For those who are not familiar with multinomial logistic regression analysis, it is basically an extension of the 'normal' logistic regression analysis. In fact, a multinomial logistic regression analysis is a sort of mixture of several logistic regression analyses, in which the different categories are compared to a 'reference' category. Therefore, as a result of multinomial logistic regression analysis, different odds ratios are obtained. When a multilevel data structure exists, also for multinomial logistic regression analysis, a multilevel extension can be applied. Suppose that, instead of the dichotomous outcome variable hyperchosterolemia, three groups are considered, i.e. a group of patients with relatively 'low' cholesterol values, a group of patients with relatively 'moderate' cholesterol values, and a group of patients with relatively 'high' cholesterol values. Again, the research question of interest is the relationship between total cholesterol and age. Output 4.7 shows the dataset used in this example.

From Output 4.7, it can be seen that the outcome variable is now called 'total cholesterol group'; and that the possible values range between 0 and 2. All other variables in the example dataset are already known from earlier examples. Output 4.8 shows the results of a 'naive' multinomial logistic multilevel analysis, in which the dependency of the observations within the medical doctors is ignored.

Output 4.8 looks a bit different from the earlier outputs. This is basically due to fact that the multinomial logistic multilevel analysis is only available in the latest version of MLwiN (Version 2.0). In the first line of Output 4.8 the outcome variable is called 'resp', which stands for *response variable*. It is

Output 4.7. Descriptive information regarding the dataset used in the example to explain multinomial logistic multilevel analysis

Name	n	missing	min	max
1 total cholesterol group	441	0	0	2
2 medical doctor	441	0	1	12
3 age	441	0	44	86
4 id	441	0	1	441
5 cons	441	0	1	1

1 total cholesterol | Refresh | Categories | Help

Output 4.8. Results of a 'naive' multinomial logistic multilevel analysis of the relationship between total cholesterol (divided into three groups) and age

$$\text{resp}_{ijk} \sim \text{Multinomial}(\text{cons}_{jk}, \pi_{ijk})$$
$$\log(\pi_{1jk}/\pi_{0jk}) = -5,629(0,698)\text{cons.moderate cholesterol}_{ijk} +$$
$$0,096(0,011)\text{age.moderate cholesterol}_{ijk}$$
$$\log(\pi_{2jk}/\pi_{0jk}) = -9,575(0,761)\text{cons.high cholesterol}_{ijk} +$$
$$0,157(0,012)\text{age.high cholesterol}_{ijk}$$
$$\text{cov}(y_{sjk}, y_{rjk}) = \pi_{sjk}\pi_{rjk}/\text{cons}_{jk}{:}s \neq r; \pi_{sjk}(1 - \pi_{rjk})/$$
$$\text{cons}_{jk}{:}s = r;$$

surprising that the response variable has three subscripts, while there are only two levels (i.e. the patient and the medical doctor). This has to do with the way MLwiN performs a multinomial logistic multilevel analysis, which is not important for the interpretation of the results, and will therefore not be discussed further. From the first line of the output it can also be seen that a multinomial logistic regression is performed, which means that the response variable must be categorical (note that the *cons* statement has exactly the same meaning as the *denom* statement in the multilevel logistic regression analysis and note that *bcons* does not have to be added). The following lines of the output show the result of the multinomial logistic multilevel analysis. The regression coefficients for age can be transformed to odds ratios by taking EXP[regression coefficient]. So, for the 'moderate cholesterol' group, the odds ratio for age is EXP[0.096] = 1.10, which means that for a difference of 1 year in age, the odds of being in the 'moderate' cholesterol group is 1.10 times higher than the odds of being in the 'low' cholesterol group. Analogue, the odds of being in the 'high' cholesterol group is EXP[0.157] = 1.17 times higher than the odds of being in the 'low' cholesterol group. The lowest line of the output contains some information regarding the multinomial logistic regression analysis, but does not provide any information that is important for the interpretation of the results, so it can therefore be ignored. The next step in the analysis is to allow a random intercept, or, in other words, the next step is to correct for the dependency of the observations within the medical doctor. In this situation, in which a categorical variable with three groups is considered as outcome variable, it indicates that two random intercepts are added to the model. Output 4.9 shows the results of a multinomial logistic multilevel analysis in which a correction is made for medical doctor, or, in other words a multinomial logistic regression analysis in which the intercept is allowed to vary among medical doctors.

Output 4.9. Results of a multinomial logistic multilevel analysis with a random intercept to determine the relationship between total cholesterol (divided into three groups) and age

$resp_{ijk} \sim \text{Multinomial}(cons_{jk}, \pi_{ijk})$

$\log(\pi_{1jk}/\pi_{0jk}) = \beta_{0k}cons.\text{moderate cholesterol}_{ijk} +$
$\qquad\qquad\qquad 0,103(0,011)age.\text{moderate cholesterol}_{ijk}$

$\beta_{0k} = -6,068(0,733) + v_{0k}$

$\log(\pi_{2jk}/\pi_{0jk}) = \beta_{1k}cons.\text{high cholesterol}_{ijk} +$
$\qquad\qquad\qquad 0,172(0,012)age.\text{high cholesterol}_{ijk}$

$\beta_{1k} = -10,492(0,872) + v_{1k}$

$\begin{bmatrix} v_{0k} \\ v_{1k} \end{bmatrix} \sim N(0, \Omega_v) : \Omega_v = \begin{bmatrix} 0,262(0,155) & \\ -0,564(0,288) & 1,392(0,620) \end{bmatrix}$

$\text{cov}(y_{sjk}, y_{rjk}) = \pi_{sjk}\pi_{rjk}/cons_{jk} : s \neq r; \pi_{sjk}(1 - \pi_{rjk})/$
$\qquad\qquad\qquad cons_{jk} : s = r;$

From Output 4.9 it can be seen that the regression coefficients (and therefore the corresponding odds ratios) are remarkably different from the ones estimated in the 'naive' analysis and shown in Output 4.8. Both regression coefficients are higher, while the standard errors remain more or less the same. So probably, the correction for medical doctor was important. This can also be seen from the variances of the two intercepts. These are shown in the variance/covariance matrix, which is shown beyond the two regression equations. The variance of the first intercept (i.e. comparing the 'low' cholesterol group with the 'moderate' cholesterol group) is 0.262, while the intercept of the second intercept (i.e. comparing the 'low' cholesterol group with the 'high' cholesterol group) is 1.392. Note that in this matrix also the covariance between the two intercepts is provided and that v_{0k} and v_{1k}, instead of u_{0k} and u_{1k} identify the variances of the intercepts. Again, this has to do with the way MLwiN performs a multinomial logistic multilevel analysis.

As in the case of logistic multilevel analysis, the necessity for allowing the intercepts to be random cannot be evaluated by the likelihood ratio test, because the regression coefficients are estimated with a quasi-likelihood procedure instead of a maximum likelihood procedure. So, the magnitude of the variances compared to their standard errors must be used to evaluate this necessity. Based on the magnitude of the variances and the standard errors, it seems to be quite reasonable to allow the intercepts to be random. Note, however, that this decision is arbitrary, because the Wald test cannot be used for variances and there is no real cut-off for the ratio between the magnitude of the variance and the standard error. The odds ratios for age, estimated from the results of the analysis that was last performed, are respectively EXP[0.103] = 1.11, with a 95% CI ranging from 1.08 to 1.13, and EXP[0.172] = 1.19, with a 95% CI ranging from 1.16 to 1.22.

A next possible step in the analysis is to allow the regression coefficients for age to be random. However, the coefficients of that model could not be estimated with the MLwiN software. So the most appropriate 'model' to estimate the relationship between age and total cholesterol (divided into three groups) was shown in Output 4.9. It should be noted that the regression coefficients presented in Outputs 4.8 and 4.9 were estimated with a first order MQL estimation procedure. As in the logistic multilevel analysis, a second order PQL estimation procedure seems to lead to 'better' results than a first order MQL procedure. However, a second order PQL estimation was

Table 4.2. Results of multinomial logistic regression analyses with different estimation procedures, with and without a random intercept

	Regression coefficient	Standard error
'Naive' analysis (maximum likelihood)		
Moderate versus low	0.104	0.017
High versus low	0.162	0.018
'Naive' analysis (quasi-likelihood)		
Moderate versus low	0.096	0.011
High versus low	0.157	0.012
Multilevel analysis (quasi-likelihood)[1]		
Moderate versus low	0.103	0.011
High versus low	0.172	0.012

[1] A 'corrected' analysis (i.e. allowing random intercepts) cannot be performed with maximum likelihood.

not possible in the situation with a random intercept. Table 4.2 summarises the results of the different analyses, in combination with the results of a 'naive' multinomial logistic multilevel analysis estimated with maximum likelihood, which can be performed with all standard software packages. Although all observed relationships are highly statistically significant, the difference in results between the different analyses also indicates the complexity of estimating the regression coefficients in these multinomial multilevel situations.

In the analyses described in this Section, 'regular' multinomial logistic multilevel analysis was performed. However, it is also possible to perform a so-called 'ordered' multinomial logistic multilevel analysis (also known as a '*proportional odds analysis*'). This analysis takes into account the ordering of the categorical outcome variable. The biggest difference, compared to 'regular' multinomial logistic multilevel analysis, is that the regression coefficients must be interpreted differently. In 'regular' multinomial logistic multilevel analysis, both the 'moderate' cholesterol group and the 'high' cholesterol group were compared to the 'low' cholesterol group separately. In an 'ordered' multinomial logistic multilevel analysis, the combined 'moderate' and 'high' cholesterol groups are compared to the 'low' cholesterol group, and the 'high' cholesterol group is compared to the 'low' cholesterol group.

Basically, instead of modelling the response probabilities of the separate categories, the cumulative response probabilities are modelled. The ordered multinomial logistic regression analysis has some slight advantages when the categories of the outcome variable are ordered (as in the present example). For instance, it can be slightly more efficient, because when the odds are proportional, only one regression coefficient (i.e. odds ratio) has to be estimated. However, the interpretation of the 'regular' multinomial logistic multilevel analysis is somewhat easier, especially for non-experienced users, and when there are not so many categories in the outcome variable. For a more detailed mathematical explanation of multinomial logistic multilevel analysis, reference is made to Daniels and Gatsonics (1997), Yang (1997), Fielding (1999), Agresti et al. (2000), Fielding (2001), Rabe-Hesketh and Skrondal (2001a), Grilli and Rampichini (2003), Skrondal and Rabe-Hesketh (2003a), and Fielding et al. (2003).

4.4 Poisson multilevel analysis

In Section 4.3, multinomial logistic multilevel analysis (i.e. multilevel analysis with a categorical outcome variable) was discussed. It should be noted that the software that is needed to perform this kind of analysis is still being developed, so the results obtained from this type of analysis must be interpreted with caution. This is different for a specific kind of categorical variable, i.e. a so-called 'count' variable (e.g. the number of physical complaints, the number of epileptic seizures, the number of asthma attacks, etc.). In fact for performing multilevel analysis on 'count' outcome variables, many different software packages are available (see also Chapter 9).

Multilevel analysis with a 'count' outcome variable is a Poisson regression analysis, in which an additional correction can be made for categorical variables (with many categories). The use of Poisson multilevel analysis, and the interpretation of the results, will be explained with an example in which the outcome variable is the number of risk factors observed in a certain patient. The number of risk factors can range from 0 to 5, and the distribution of this variable in the example population is shown in Figure 4.1.

Output 4.10 gives the descriptive information regarding this example with a 'count' outcome variable. In the first line of Output 4.10 it can be seen

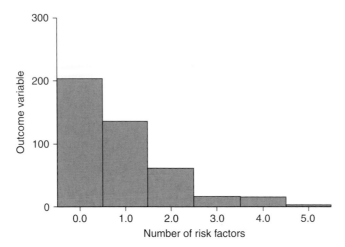

Figure 4.1. The distribution of the number of risk factor: the outcome variable used to explain Poisson multilevel analysis.

Output 4.10. Descriptive information regarding the dataset used in the example to explain Poisson multilevel analysis

	Name	n	missing	min	max	
1	**number of risk factors**	441	0	0	5	
2	medical doctor	441	0	1	12	
3	age	441	0	44	86	
4	id	441	0	1	441	
5	cons	441	0	1	1	
6	bcons	441	0	1	1	

(window: 1 number of risk | | | Refresh | Categories | Help)

that the number of risk factors can vary between 0 and 5. There are again 12 medical doctors and the age of the patients still ranges between 44 and 86 years. Note that, as in logistic multilevel analysis, in Poisson multilevel analysis a *bcons* column is also needed. The reason for this is the same as for dichotomous outcome variables.

Output 4.11 shows the results of a 'naive' Poisson multilevel analysis, i.e. ignoring the dependency of the observations within medical doctors.

Output 4.11. Results of a 'naive' Poisson multilevel analysis of the relationship between the number of risk factors and age

$$
\begin{aligned}
&\text{number of risk factors}_{ij} \sim \text{Poisson}(\pi_{ij}) \\
&\text{number of risk factors}_{ij} = \pi_{ij} + e_{0ij}\text{bcons}^*
\end{aligned}
$$

$$\log(\pi_{ij}) = -1{,}566\,(0{,}336)\,\text{cons} + 0{,}023\,(0{,}005)\,\text{age}_{ij}$$

$$\text{bcons}^* = \text{bcons}\ \pi_{ij}^{0.5}$$

$$[e_{0ij}] \sim (0,\ \Omega_e)\ :\ \Omega_e = [1{,}000\,(0{,}000)]$$

Output 4.11 looks similar to the outputs described earlier for linear and logistic multilevel analysis. The first line of the output shows that the outcome variable (i.e. number of risk factors) is a Poisson outcome variable, and in the second line the 'error variance' is defined (see for the explanation of this 'error variance' Section 4.2, in which the 'error variance' was explained for logistic multilevel analysis). The third line of the output shows the actual Poisson regression model. First of all, it can be seen that the logarithm of the outcome variable is used (that is also the reason why Poisson regression analysis is sometimes called log linear regression analysis). Furthermore, it can be seen that the regression coefficient for age is 0.023, with a standard error of 0.005. This regression coefficient can be transformed into a 'rate ratio' by taking EXP[regression coefficient]. In the present example this 'rate ratio' equals 1.02, with a 95% CI ranging from 1.01 to 1.03. The 'rate ratio' of 1.02 can be interpreted in such a way that a difference of 1 year in age is associated with 1.02 times more risk factors. As for the odds ratio calculated from a logistic multilevel analysis, the 'rate ratio' is also small with a narrow 95% CI. This is again due to the scale in which the independent age variable is measured. However, this result also implies that a difference of 10 years of age is associated with EXP[10×0.023] = 1.22 (or $(1.02)^{10} = 1.22$) times more risk factors, or a 22% increase in the number of risk factors. The last two lines of the output are related to the fact that a Poisson regression analysis is performed, and since this information is not really important for the interpretation of the results it will not be discussed.

Output 4.12 shows the output of a Poisson regression analysis in which a correction is made for medical doctor. Or, in other words, a Poisson regression analysis in which the intercept is allowed to vary between medical doctors.

Output 4.12. Results of a Poisson multilevel analysis with a random intercept to determine the relationship between the number of risk factors and age

$$
\begin{aligned}
&\texttt{number of risk factors}_{ij} ~ \texttt{Poisson}(\pi_{ij})\\
&\texttt{number of risk factors}_{ij} = \pi_{ij} + e_{0ij}\texttt{bcons}^*
\end{aligned}
\left.\phantom{\begin{aligned}&\\&\end{aligned}}\right\}
$$

$\log(\pi_{ij}) = \beta_{1j}\texttt{cons} + 0,024(0,005)\texttt{age}_{ij}$

$\beta_{1j} = -1,599(0,362) + u_{1j}$

$[u_{1j}] ~ N(0, \Omega_u) : \Omega_u = [0,145(0,071)]$

$\texttt{bcons}^* = \texttt{bcons}\ \pi_{ij}^{0,5}$

$[e_{0ij}] ~ (0, \Omega_e) : \Omega_e = [1,000(0,000)]$

The fact that a random intercept is added to the analysis can be seen in the fourth line of Output 4.12, which shows the value of the intercept and the (random) variance of this intercept (again coded as u_{1j}). The value of this variance (i.e. 0.145) and the corresponding standard error (i.e. 0.071) are shown in the next line of the output. As for the logistic multilevel analysis, the parameters from the Poisson multilevel analysis are estimated with quasi-likelihood, and therefore, the -2 log likelihood can not be estimated. So, the likelihood ratio test cannot be used to evaluate the necessity of assuming a random intercept. Therefore, also for Poisson multilevel analysis, the necessity of allowing random regression coefficients (i.e. a random intercept) can be evaluated from the magnitude of the variance and the corresponding standard error. In the example, the ratio of the variance and the standard error is 2.04, suggesting that a random intercept is probably necessary. Again, it is statistically not correct to do so, but in practice it is probably one of the only possibilities to get some idea of the necessity of allowing random regression coefficients. Again, there is no real cut-off value that can be used, so the decision with regard to whether or not to allow a random regression coefficient is always arbitrary.

The second step in the analysis can be to also allow the regression coefficient for age to vary among medical doctors (i.e. allowing a random slope for age). Output 4.13 shows the result of this analysis.

Output 4.13. Results of a Poisson multilevel analysis with a random intercept and a random slope for age to determine the relationship between the number of risk factors and age

$$\left. \begin{array}{l} \text{number of risk factors}_{ij} ~ \sim~ \texttt{Poisson}(\pi_{ij}) \\ \text{number of risk factors}_{ij} ~=~ \pi_{ij} ~+~ e_{0ij}\texttt{bcons}^* \end{array} \right\}$$

$$\log(\pi_{ij}) ~=~ \beta_{1j}\texttt{cons} ~+~ \beta_{2j}\texttt{age}_{ij}$$

$$\beta_{1j} ~=~ -1,37408\,(0,66047) ~+~ u_{1j}$$

$$\beta_{2j} ~=~ 0,02052\,(0,01087) ~+~ u_{2j}$$

$$\begin{bmatrix} u_{1j} \\ u_{2j} \end{bmatrix} \sim N(0,~\Omega_u) ~:~ \Omega_u ~=~ \begin{bmatrix} 3,52220(2,09805) & \\ -0,05810(0,03422) & 0,00099(0,00057) \end{bmatrix}$$

$$\texttt{bcons}^* ~=~ \texttt{bcons}~\pi_{ij}^{0.5}$$

$$[e_{0ij}] ~\sim~ (0,~\Omega_e) ~:~ \Omega_e ~=~ [1,00000\,(0,00000)]$$

From Output 4.13 it can be seen that a variance is added to the regression coefficient for age (i.e. u_{2j} is added to the model). The magnitude of the variance of the regression coefficient for age is 0.00099, with a standard error of 0.00057. The ratio between the two is therefore 1.74, and although this value is less than 2, the random variance of the regression coefficient for age may be considered to be important. Another (alternative) way in which to evaluate whether or not a random regression coefficient 'must' be allowed is to compare the regression coefficients in a model with and a model without the random regression coefficient. If the regression coefficient for age is compared in the analysis with and the analysis without the random slope for age, it can be seen that both the regression coefficient and the standard error are remarkably different. This difference can be used as an argument that a random slope should probably be considered. However, it should be realised that all arguments for or against adding a random regression coefficient to a Poisson multilevel regression model are rather arbitrary. From Output 4.13 it can also be seen that the covariance between the random intercept and the random slope for age has a negative sign, which implies that when a high intercept is observed for a particular medical doctor, the relationship between the number of risk factors and age is less strong.

As in the case of logistic multilevel analysis various estimation procedures are also available for Poisson multilevel analysis. In the examples presented in this section, a first order MQL estimation procedure was used. Although the analysis was not very complicated, it was not possible to use a second order PQL estimation procedure (i.e. the model did not converge, or, in other words, did not lead to a valid result).

A more mathematical discussion of Poisson multilevel analysis can be found, for instance, in Christiansen and Morris (1997), Albert and Follman (2000).

4.5 Multilevel survival analysis

In Section 4.2 a logistic multilevel analysis was discussed. Logistic multilevel analysis can be used to analyse a dichotomous outcome variable, and in the example the dichotomous outcome variable hypercholesterolemia was the 'event' of interest. When the data in a study provide not only information about whether the 'event' of interest occurs in a patient, but also at what point in time it occurs, this additional information can be included in the analysis by applying survival analysis, i.e. Cox (proportional hazards) regression analysis. In Cox-regression analysis both the occurrence of the event and the time when the patient was at risk for the occurrence of that event are used as outcome variable. Due to the hazard function over time is modelled in Cox-regression analysis, the result of such an analysis is a hazard ratio. At present, the only software in which multilevel Cox-regression analysis can be performed is implemented in the General Linear Latent and Mixed Models (gllamm) procedure in STATA (see Chapter 9). However, this procedure is far from straightforward, and it goes beyond the scope of this book to explain it in detail (see for details Rabe-Hesketh et al., 2004; Chapter 7). One of the reasons for this complexity is probably the fact that there is no 'real' intercept in a Cox-regression model. There is an intercept, but because it can be seen as the 'baseline hazard function' it changes over time.

In MLwiN there are also some possibilities to perform a type of survival analysis. However, this is only possible with syntax macros, and the analyses that can be performed do not answer the questions that can be answered with 'standard' Cox-regression analyses (see for details Goldstein, 1995; Yang et al., 1999; Leyland et al., 2000; Goldstein, 2003). For more mathematical details, reference is made, for instance, to Ten Have (1996), Hogan and Laird (1997). Sastry (1997), Schieke and Jensen (1997), Barthelemy (2001), Merlo et al. (2001), Vaida and Xu (2001), Yau (2001), and Xu and Zeger (2001). So, what can be done when not only survival data is available in a study, but when that data is also clustered, for instance, within medical doctors? In several software packages (e.g. STATA and SPSS) there is an additional option for the Cox-regression analysis that allows the baseline hazard functions to differ between strata. This analysis can therefore be seen as a 'primitive' multilevel survival analysis, in which a random intercept is considered. Let us go back to the example discussed in Section 4.1. In this example the relationship between the dichotomous outcome variable hypercholesterolemia and age was analysed. Suppose that the study population consisted of a certain cohort of individuals, free from hypercholesterolemia at baseline, and suppose also that there was a maximum follow-up of 5 years, and that both the occurrence of hypercholesterolemia and the time when it occurred were registered. The research question is still the same: what is the relationship between the occurrence of hypercholesterolemia and age (which is now the age at baseline in the study). Table 4.3 shows descriptive information regarding this example dataset.

Compared to the descriptive information regarding the example used in Section 4.1 (see Output 4.1) the follow-up period is added to the dataset. It can be seen that the follow-up period ranges between 3 and 60 months. The latter is the maximum number of months, because the total follow-up period of the study was 5 years. Ignoring the fact that the observations are clustered within the medical doctor, a 'naive' Cox-regression analysis can be performed, with age as the only independent variable. Output 4.14 shows the results of this 'naive' Cox-regression analysis performed in STATA.

Table 4.3. Descriptive information regarding the dataset used for the 'multilevel' Cox-regression analysis

	Number	Minimum	Maximum
Hypercholesterolemia	441	0	1
Medical doctor	441	1	12
Age	441	44	86
follow-up period (months)	441	3	60

Output 4.14. Results of a 'naive' Cox-regression analysis of the relationship between time to hypercholesterolemia and age performed in STATA

```
No. of subjects  =           441         Number of obs   =        441
No. of failures  =           171
Time at risk     =         17610
                                         LR chi2(1)      =      37.35
Log likelihood   =  -903.15952          Prob > chi2     =     0.0000
------------------------------------------------------------------------
  _t |
  _d |  Haz. Ratio  Std. Err.   z    P>|z|  [95% Conf. Interval]
-----+------------------------------------------------------------------
 age |  1.049109    .0081099  6.20  0.000  1.033334    1.065125
------------------------------------------------------------------------
```

The first part of Output 4.14 provides some general information about the analysis. It can be seen that there are 441 observations, there are 171 subjects with hypercholesterolemia (i.e. the prevalence of hypercholesterolemia was 39%), and the total follow-up period for the entire study population is 17,610 months. Furthermore, the log likelihood of this model is shown (-903.15952), and the significance of the 'total' model (i.e. in this situation the model with one independent variable age), compared to a model without independent variables. The model with age is significantly better than the model without age, so age is significantly related to the occurrence of hypercholesterolemia and/or the time of that occurrence. The magnitude of the relationship can be seen in the last part of the output, which shows a hazard ratio of 1.049109. This means that for a difference of 1 year in age, the hazard of developing hypercholesterolemia increases with 1.049109. Although the absolute value of the hazard ratio is quite low, it is highly significant ($z = 6.20$ and the corresponding p-value is <0.001). Again, the reason for the relatively low magnitude of the hazard ratio is that age is given in years, and that a difference of 1 year is a very small difference. It is more appropriate to show the hazard ratio for a bigger difference in age. So, for instance, the hazard ratio for a difference of 10 years in age is $(1.049109)^{10} = 1.62$. To obtain a 95% CI around this hazard ratio, the same procedure must be followed with the shown CI for a difference of 1 year in age. It should again be noted that because the intercept (i.e. the baseline hazard function) changes over time, no intercept is shown in the output.

To correct for the dependency of the observations within medical doctors a so-called stratified Cox-regression analysis can be performed. Output 4.15 shows the results of such an analysis.

Output 4.15. Results of a stratified Cox-regression analysis of the relationship between time to hypercholesterolemia and age performed in STATA

```
No. of subjects   =          441          Number of obs   =        441
No. of failures   =          171
Time at risk      =        17610
                                           LR chi2(1)      =      24.67
Log likelihood    =   -485.28636           Prob > chi2     =     0.0000
-----------------------------------------------------------------------
   _t |
   _d |   Haz. Ratio  Std. Err.   z     P>|z|   [95% Conf. Interval]
--------+--------------------------------------------------------------
  age |   1.045717    .0096389   4.85  0.000   1.026995    1.064781
-----------------------------------------------------------------------
                                           Stratified by medical doctor
```

The last line of Output 4.15 shows that the analysis is *stratified by medical doctor*. This means that the baseline hazard functions are allowed to differ between medical doctors, or, in other words, the 'intercept' is allowed to differ between medical doctors. To evaluate whether this 'random intercept' is necessary, the likelihood ratio test can be applied. With this test the $-2\log$ likelihood of the two models (i.e. with and without a random 'intercept') must be compared. The difference between the $-2\log$ likelihood of the two models is huge ($2 \times (903.15952 - 485.28636) = 835.7$). This difference, however, does not follow a Chi-square distribution with one degree of freedom, which is due to the fact that the stratified Cox-regression analysis is not a 'real' multilevel analysis. In the stratified Cox-regression analysis, it is not the variance of the different baseline hazard functions that is estimated, but all baseline hazard functions for the different medical doctors are estimated. So, instead of one baseline hazard function in the 'naive' Cox-regression analysis, 12 baseline hazard functions are estimated in the stratified Cox-regression analysis. In other words, the difference in $-2\log$ likelihood of the two models must be evaluated on a Chi-square distribution with 11 degrees of freedom (which is nevertheless highly significant). The influence of allowing different baseline hazard functions for the medical doctors is that the hazard ratio for age is slightly lower, while the standard error (and therefore the width of the 95% CI) is slightly higher.

The results presented in Output 4.15 provide the final result of this analysis, because with a stratified Cox-regression analysis it is not possible to allow the regression coefficients for age to differ between medical doctors. In other words, the hazard ratio for age is 1.046, with a 95% CI ranging from 1.027 to 1.065.

It should be noted that exactly the same results could be obtained from a stratified Cox-regression analysis performed in SPSS.

5

Multilevel modelling

5.1 Introduction

Up to now, the explanation of the principles of multilevel analysis has been limited to simple analysis. In this chapter, the models to be analysed will be extended with some covariates. Let us go back to the result of one of the analyses performed in Chapter 2 (see Output 2.5). In this analysis a two-level structure was considered, in such a way that patients were clustered within medical doctors (see Figure 2.4), and the relationship between age and total cholesterol was investigated. The independent age variable was centred in order to facilitate the interpretation of the (variance of the random) intercept when a random slope for age was allowed. The example with age centred is chosen as a starting point because the magnitude of the variance of the random intercept is going to be used in the next part of this section. The conclusion of the analysis performed in Chapter 2 was that there was a highly significant positive relationship between age and total cholesterol. It was further shown that in the two-level data structure in which the patients were only clustered within the medical doctors, the 'best' way to analyse this relationship was a model with a random intercept as well as a random slope for age at the medical doctor level. Output 5.1 shows (again) the results of this analysis, which is used as starting point for the explanation of multilevel modelling.

5.2 Multivariable multilevel analysis

Suppose that it is believed that body mass index (BMI) plays a role in this relationship, and therefore a correction is made for BMI. Output 5.2 shows the dataset, in which BMI is added, and for a better interpretation of the magnitude of the intercept, BMI is also centred.

Output 5.1. Results of a linear multilevel analysis of the relationship between total cholesterol and age with both a random intercept and a random slope for age at the medical doctor level, when age is centred

```
total cholesterol_ij ~ N(XB, Ω)

total cholesterol_ij = β_0ij cons + β_1j age_centred_ij
β_0ij = 5,97120(0,17562) + u_0j + e_0ij
β_1j = 0,05006(0,00576) + u_1j
```

$$\begin{bmatrix} u_{0j} \\ u_{1j} \end{bmatrix} \sim N(0, \ \Omega_u) \ : \ \Omega_u = \begin{bmatrix} 0,36113\,(0,15111) \\ -0,00036(0,00350) & 0,00027(0,00016) \end{bmatrix}$$

$$[e_{0ij}] \sim N(0, \ \Omega_e) \ : \ \Omega_e = [0,31367(0,02171)]$$

```
-2*loglikelihood(IGLS) = 799,96340(441 of 441 cases in use)
```

Output 5.2. Descriptive information regarding the example dataset including BMI

6 bmi_centred		Refresh	Categories	? Help

Name	n	missing	min	max	▲
1 total cholesterol	441	0	3,9	8,86	
2 medical doctor	441	0	1	12	
3 age	441	0	44	86	
4 age_centred	441	0	-17,7551	24,2449	
5 bmi	441	0	20,2	44,05	
6 bmi_centred	441	0	-11,0174	12,8326	
7 id	441	0	1	441	
8 cons	441	0	1	1	▼

From the descriptive information it can be seen that the BMI of the patients range between 20.20 and 44.05. All other variables are the same as in the earlier examples. Output 5.3 shows the results of the linear multilevel analysis of the relationship between age and total cholesterol corrected for BMI (i.e. the centred value of BMI).

Output 5.3. Results of a linear multilevel analysis of the relationship between total cholesterol and age, with both a random intercept and a random slope for age at the medical doctor level, when age is centred, corrected for BMI (centred)

```
total cholesterolᵢⱼ ~ N(XB, Ω)
total cholesterolᵢⱼ = β₀ᵢⱼcons + β₁ⱼage_centredᵢⱼ +
                      0,03370(0,00591)bmi_centredᵢⱼ
β₀ᵢⱼ = 5,97126(0,15138) + u₀ⱼ + e₀ᵢⱼ
β₁ⱼ = 0,04807(0,00506) + u₁ⱼ
```

$$\begin{bmatrix} u_{0j} \\ u_{1j} \end{bmatrix} \sim N(0, \Omega_u) : \Omega_u = \begin{bmatrix} 0{,}26657(0{,}11221) & \\ -0{,}00114(0{,}00266) & 0{,}00019(0{,}00012) \end{bmatrix}$$

```
[e₀ᵢⱼ] ~ N(0, Ωₑ) : Ωₑ = [0,29622(0,02051)]

-2*loglikelihood(IGLS) = 769,29660(441 of 441 cases in use)
```

From Output 5.3 it can be seen that BMI is highly significant related to total cholesterol. The Wald statistic is $(0.03370/0.00591)^2 = 32.52$, which is Chi-square distributed with one degree of freedom; i.e. the p-value < 0.001. However, the relationship between age and total cholesterol did not change a lot by adding BMI to the model. The regression coefficient for age changed from 0.050 to 0.048. In other words, the relationship between age and total cholesterol is not (or hardly) influenced by BMI. On the other hand, it can also be seen that the magnitude of the variances of the random intercept and the random slope decreased remarkably when BMI was added to the model. The variance of the random intercept decreased from 0.36113 to 0.26657 and the variance of the random slope decreased from 0.00027 to 0.00019. So, presumably part of the differences between medical doctors can be explained by the BMI of the patient. So, in general it is possible to 'explain' the random variance in either the intercept or the slopes by certain covariates.

BMI is a variable that is measured at patient level, but it can also be interesting to analyse the additional value of variables that are measured at the medical doctor level. Suppose we have some additional information of the medical doctors, e.g. the age of the medical doctor (see Output 5.4).

Output 5.4. Descriptive information regarding the example dataset including BMI and the age of the medical doctor

10 md_centred			Refresh	Categories	? Help	
Name	**n**		**missing**	**min**	**max**	
1 total cholesterol	441		0	3,9	8,86	
2 medical doctor	441		0	1	12	
3 age	441		0	44	86	
4 age_centred	441		0	-17,7551	24,2449	
5 bmi	441		0	20,2	44,05	
6 bmi_centred	441		0	-11,0174	12,8326	
7 id	441		0	1	441	
8 cons	441		0	1	1	
9 age medical doctor	441		0	40	55	
10 age md_centred	441		0	-4,224499	10,7755	

From Output 5.4 it can be seen that the age range of the medical doctors is between 40 and 55 years. Output 5.5 shows the results of an analysis in which the age of the medical doctor (also centred) is added to the regression model that was shown in Output 5.1.

Output 5.5. Results of a linear multilevel analysis of the relationship between total cholesterol and age, with both a random intercept and a random slope for age at the medical doctor level, when age is centred, corrected for the age of the medical doctor (centred)

$$\text{total cholesterol}_{ij} \sim N(XB, \ \Omega)$$
$$\text{total cholesterol}_{ij} = \beta_{0ij}\text{cons} + \beta_{1j}\text{age\_centred}_{ij} +$$
$$0,12811(0,02318)\text{age md\_centred}_j$$
$$\beta_{0ij} = 5,96804(0,09451) + u_{0j} + e_{0ij}$$
$$\beta_{1j} = 0,05016(0,00577) + u_{1j}$$

$$\begin{vmatrix} u_{0j} \\ u_{1j} \end{vmatrix} \sim N(0, \ \Omega_u) \ : \ \Omega_u = \begin{bmatrix} 0,09821(0,04377) \\ 0,00077(0,00190) & 0,00027(0,00016) \end{bmatrix}$$
$$[e_{0ij}] \sim N(0, \ \Omega_e) \ : \ \Omega_e = [0,31357(0,02171)]$$

$$-2*loglikelihood(IGLS) = 784,86120(441 \text{ of } 441 \text{ cases in use})$$

From Output 5.5 it can be seen that the age of the medical doctor is highly related to total cholesterol values of the patient. The Wald statistic is $(0.12811/0.02318)^2 = 30.54$, which corresponds with a p-value < 0.001. However, adding age of the medical doctor to the model does not influence the relationship between age (of the patient) and total cholesterol. On the other hand, the addition of the age of the medical doctor to the model has resulted in a huge reduction in the variance of the random intercept on the medical doctor level (the variance decreased from 0.36113 to 0.09821). From this huge reduction in the variance, it can be concluded that a great amount of the differences between medical doctors is caused by the different ages of the medical doctors. The variance of the slopes (i.e. the difference in the relationship between age and total cholesterol between medical doctors) on the other hand is not influenced by the age of the medical doctor.

So, the addition of covariates to the multilevel model give: (1) Information whether or not a certain covariate is a confounder in the relationship of interest. This is exactly the same as in 'standard' (linear) regression analysis, and can be evaluated by the difference in the regression coefficient of interest between a model with and a model without the covariate. (2) Information whether certain variables explain the difference observed in higher level groups (e.g. medical doctors). The latter is (of course) a special feature of using multilevel analysis.

In the same way as described above also interaction terms can be added to the multilevel models. An interaction term (i.e. a multiplication of the variable of interest (i.e. age of the patient) and the potential effect modifier) is added to analyse whether the observed relationship between age and total cholesterol is different for different groups of the potential effect modifier. The way this is done in multilevel analysis is exactly the same as this is done in 'standard' (linear) regression analysis. A special feature of multilevel analysis is that so-called 'cross-level' interactions can be analysed. A cross-level interaction indicates that an interaction between a variable measured on the lower level and a variable measured on a higher level is added to the regression model. The way this is done in multilevel analysis is exactly the same as for 'normal' interaction terms. In the example we can, for instance, be interested in the cross-level interaction between age of the patient and the age of the medical doctor. Output 5.6 shows the results of the analysis that includes this cross-level interaction.

Output 5.6. Results of a linear multilevel analysis of the relationship between total cholesterol and age, with both a random intercept and a random slope for age at the medical doctor level, when age is centred, corrected for the age of the medical doctor (centred) and including the interaction between age (of the patient) and the age of the medical doctor

```
total cholesterol_ij ~ N(XB, Ω)
total cholesterol_ij = β_0ij cons + β_1j age_centred_ij +
                       0,12706(0,02333)age md_centred_j +
                       -0,00049(0,00139)interaction_age_ageMD_ij
β_0ij = 5,96824(0,09435) + u_0j + e_0ij
β_1j = 0,05017(0,00574) + u_1j
```

$$
\begin{bmatrix} u_{0j} \\ u_{1j} \end{bmatrix} \sim N(0, \; \Omega_u) \; : \; \Omega_u = \begin{bmatrix} 0,09784(0,04362) & \\ 0,00070(0,00189) & 0,00027(0,00016) \end{bmatrix}
$$

$$[e_{0ij}] \sim N(0, \; \Omega_e) \; : \; \Omega_e = [0,31358(0,02171)]$$

```
-2*loglikelihood(IGLS) = 784,73950(441 of 441 cases in use)
```

From Output 5.6 it can be seen that the interaction between age (of the patient) and age of the medical doctor is not statistically significant. The Wald statistic for the interaction is $(-0.00048/0.00139)^2 = 0.12$, which gives a p-value of 0.729. When a cross-level interaction is added to the analysis, it is also interesting to look at the change in the variance of the random slope. It is possible that part of the differences in the regression coefficient for age (of the patient) between medical doctors is caused by the difference in the ages of the medical doctors. In this example, there is, however, no influence on the random slope, because the variance of the slope derived from a model without the interaction is exactly the same as the variance of the slope derived from a model with the interaction.

5.3 Prediction models and association models

5.3.1 Introduction

When performing a multivariable analysis, it is extremely important to realise what kind of question should be answered with the multivariable analysis. This not only applies to multivariable multilevel analysis, but basically to all multivariable analyses. Within multivariable analysis, a distinction should be made between 'prediction' or 'prognostic' models and 'association' models. With association models (see Section 5.3.2) the research question of interest concerns the association between one main or central independent variable (or a small set of central independent variables) and a certain outcome. The general idea behind association models is to estimate this relationship or association as 'accurately' as possible. This means that correction for confounding and/or possible effect modification must be taken into account. For prediction or prognostic models (Section 5.3.3) the research question (and therefore the modelling strategy) is different. Constructing a prediction model concerns searching for the best, most simple combination of independent variables to predict a certain outcome. It should be realised that each of the modelling strategies applied in the following sections of this chapter are examples of possible strategies. There are many more roads that lead to Rome!

5.3.2 Association models

The example used throughout this book, and the modelling described in Section 5.2, is basically constructing an association model. The main or central determinant in the analysis was age, and the relationship between age and total cholesterol was controlled for BMI and, in a separate analysis for the age of the medical doctor. In fact, the way association models are constructed within multilevel analysis is more or less the same as the way in which association models are constructed in 'standard' regression analysis. Probably the most common example of constructing an association model is when the effect of a certain intervention is evaluated. The main or central determinant is the intervention, and the effect of this central determinant has to be estimated as 'accurate' as possible. This means that, when necessary, the effect of the intervention has to be corrected for potential confounders, and that possible effect modification has to be taken into account. Therefore, in this section a randomised controlled trial (RCT) will be used as an example for the construction of association models. The intervention is applied with the intention of lowering total cholesterol values. The intervention is applied at the patient level, and the patients are randomly allocated into the intervention group and a control group; 131 patients were allocated to the intervention group and 145 to the control group. The patients were measured at baseline (before the start of the intervention) and directly after the intervention ended. Output 5.7 shows the descriptive information regarding the dataset used in this example.

Output 5.7. Descriptive information regarding the example dataset used to illustrate the construction of an association model

	Name	n	missing	min	max
3	intervention		Refresh	Categories	Help
1	total cholesterol	276	0	4	8,82
2	total cholesterol base	276	0	4,25	9,07
3	intervention	276	0	0	1
4	medical doctor	276	0	1	10
5	age	276	0	24	54
6	bmi	276	0	20,2	44,05
7	smoking	276	0	0	1
8	gender	276	0	0	1
9	id	276	0	1	276
10	cons	276	0	1	1

From Output 5.7 it can be seen that there are 10 medical doctors involved in the study. In addition to the outcome variable of total cholesterol (measured directly after the intervention period), there is also information available with regard to the baseline value of total cholesterol (*total cholesterol base*), and (baseline values of) age, BMI, smoking behaviour, and gender.

The first step in the construction of an association model is to perform a 'crude' analysis. In a 'crude' analysis, only the main/central determinant (i.e. the intervention variable) is present in the model. However, in the analysis of the effect of a certain intervention (evaluated in an RCT) it is important to correct for possible differences in the outcome variable at baseline (Twisk and Proper, 2004). This analysis, which is known as 'analysis of covariance' is necessary to correct for the phenomenon of 'regression to the mean', which can occur when the intervention group and the control group differ from each other with respect to the outcome variable measured at baseline. Output 5.8 shows the result of the 'naive' analysis, i.e. the analysis in which the dependency of observations within the medical doctors is ignored.

Output 5.8. Results of a 'naive' multilevel analysis to estimate the effect of the cholesterol-lowering intervention, corrected for the baseline cholesterol level

---

```
total cholesterol_ij ~ N(XB, Ω)
total cholesterol_ij = β_0i cons + 0,661(0,045)total cholesterol base_ij +
                       -0,191(0,084)intervention_ij

β_0i = 1,863(0,288) + e_0ij
[e_0ij] ~ N(0, Ω_e)  :  Ω_e = [0,484(0,041)]

-2*loglikelihood(IGLS) = 583,015(276 of 276 cases in use)
```

From Output 5.8 it can be seen that the intervention effect is -0.191. So, given a certain baseline value, the cholesterol values of the intervention group are (on average) 0.191 mmol lower than those of the control group at the follow-up measurement after the intervention. The 95% confidence interval (CI) around this effect can be calculated in the usual way, i.e. the regression coefficient ± 1.96 times the standard error. In this example the 95% CI ranges from -0.36 to -0.03. Because this interval does not include zero, the intervention effect is statistically significant. The actual p-value of the intervention effect can be derived from the Wald statistic, i.e. $(-0.191/0.084)^2 = 5.17$, which corresponds with a p-value of 0.023.

Because this significant intervention effect is derived from a 'naive' analysis, the next step in the analysis is to investigate whether or not random regression coefficients must be considered. Output 5.9 shows the results of a 'crude' multilevel analysis in which a random intercept is added to the model.

Based on the likelihood ratio test it can be seen that it is important to 'correct' for medical doctor in this analysis, i.e. it is important to add a random

Output 5.9. Results of a multilevel analysis to estimate the effect of the cholesterol-lowering intervention with a random intercept, corrected for the baseline cholesterol level

---

```
total cholesterol_ij ~ N(XB, Ω)
total cholesterol_ij = β_0ij cons + 0,473(0,052)total cholesterol base_ij +
                       -0,045(0,084)intervention_ij
β_0ij = 3,006(0,344) + u_0j + e_0ij

[u_0j]  ~ N(0, Ω_u)  :  Ω_u = [0,094(0,049)]
[e_0ij] ~ N(0, Ω_e)  :  Ω_e = [0,426(0,037)]

-2*loglikelihood(IGLS) = 567,480(276 of 276 cases in use)
```

---

intercept to the model. The difference between the two -2 log likelihoods is 15.534, which is highly significant. More important, however, is the huge reduction in the regression coefficient for the intervention variable. This coefficient decreased from -0.191 to -0.045. In fact, the intervention effect is no longer significant. The Wald statistic is $(-0.045/0.084)^2 = 0.287$, which corresponds with a p-value of 0.592.

The next step in the analysis is to add a random slope for the intervention variable to the model. Because the intervention is performed at patient level, a random slope for the intervention variable is possible. It should be realised, however, that in a study in which the randomisation is performed at the medical doctor level, a random slope for the intervention variable would not have been possible (see Section 2.8.1). Output 5.10 shows the results of this analysis.

Output 5.10. Results of a multilevel analysis to estimate the effect of the cholesterol-lowering intervention, with a random intercept and a random slope for the intervention variable, corrected for the baseline cholesterol level

```
total cholesterol_ij ~ N(XB, Ω)
total cholesterol_ij = β_0ij cons + 0,306(0,053)total cholesterol base_ij +
                       β_2j intervention_ij
β_0ij = 4,047(0,385) + u_0j + e_0ij
β_2j = -0,075(0,211) + u_2j

|u_0j|  ~ N(0, Ω_u) :  Ω_u = | 0,380(0,181)                |
|u_2j|                        |-0,370(0,183)  0,388(0,198) |
[e_0ij] ~ N(0, Ω_e) :  Ω_e = [0,350(0,031)]

-2*loglikelihood(IGLS) = 528,239(276 of 276 cases in use)
```

Based on the likelihood ratio test it can be concluded that a random slope for the intervention variable is also important. The difference between the -2 log likelihoods is 39.241, which is (evaluated on a Chi-square distribution with 2 degrees of freedom) highly significant. The intervention effect in the last analysis increased slightly, to -0.075, but because the standard error also increased, the estimated intervention effect is far from significant. The Wald statistic is $(-0.075/0.211)^2 = 0.13$, which corresponds with a p-value of 0.718. A possible next step in the analysis is to add a random slope for the baseline value of total cholesterol to the model. However, the analysis did not lead to a valid result, so the final 'crude' intervention effect can be derived from Output 5.10.

The second step in the construction procedure is to correct for (all) potential confounders. However, it should be borne in mind that in a situation in which there are many potential confounders, in comparison to the number of patients in the study, an analysis with all potential confounders is impossible. In this type of situation only important confounders can be added. The importance of a potential confounder is often evaluated on the basis of the change in the magnitude of the regression coefficient of the main or central determinant. The greater the change, the more important that potential confounder is. It is sometimes argued that only potential confounders that are associated with a change of 10% or more in the magnitude of the regression coefficient should be added to the final 'corrected' model. However, this cut-off value is highly arbitrary. The difference between multilevel analysis and 'standard' regression analysis in this second step of the construction procedure is the fact that in multilevel analysis the necessity of random regression coefficients can also be evaluated for the potential confounders. Output 5.11 shows the results of the analysis correcting for all potential confounders present in the example dataset (age, BMI, smoking and gender) without allowing the regression coefficients of the potential confounders to be random.

From Output 5.11 it can be seen that the correction for all potential covariates has some influence on the magnitude of the intervention effect. The effect changes from -0.075 to -0.119, and although the magnitude of

Output 5.11. Results of a multilevel analysis to estimate the effect of the cholesterol-lowering intervention, with a random intercept and a random slope for the intervention variable, corrected for the baseline cholesterol level, age, BMI, smoking, and gender

```
total cholesterol_ij ~ N(XB, Ω)
total cholesterol_ij = β_0ij cons + 0,215(0,050)total cholesterol base_ij +
                       β_2j intervention_ij + 0,044(0,008)age_ij +
                       0,043(0,011)bmi_ij + 0,276(0,113)smoking_ij +
                       -0,066(0,114)gender_ij

β_0ij = 1,454(0,513) + u_0j + e_0ij
β_2j  = -0,119(0,116) + u_2j

[u_0j]                      [0,242(0,117)                      ]
[u_2j] ~ N(0, Ω_u) : Ω_u =  [-0,121(0,073)  0,082(0,057)      ]

[e_0ij] ~ N(0, Ω_e) : Ω_e = [0,282(0,025)]

-2*loglikelihood(IGLS) = 467,216(276 of 276 cases in use)
```

the standard error decreases from 0.211 to 0.116, the effect is still not significant (the p-value $= 0.306$). It has been mentioned before that one of the features of multilevel analysis is that the regression coefficients of the potential confounders can also be considered random. However, this does not often happen in practice.

When reporting the results of an intervention study or in general an association model, it is strongly recommended that the results of both the 'crude' and the 'adjusted' analysis are reported. Table 5.1 shows the results of the analyses performed on the example dataset.

From Table 5.1 it can be seen that no information is provided about the random variance of the intercept and the random variance of the slope of the intervention variable. This is not strange, because we are only interested in the effect of the intervention. The reason for using multilevel analysis is that we wanted to take into account the correlated observations within the medical doctor in the most efficient way. It should be noted that the recommendation to report both the 'crude' and the 'adjusted' results does not only apply to multilevel analysis, but also for all other statistical techniques.

Another important aspect in the construction of association models is the evaluation of potential effect modification. It can, for instance, be important to determine whether the intervention effect is different for males and females. Potential effect modification can be investigated by adding interaction terms to the statistical model. An interaction term consists of a multiplication of the main/central determinant and the potential effect modifier. To investigate potential effect modification in the example dataset, we go back to the results of the 'crude' analysis that were presented in Output 5.10. In general, the way to investigate potential effect modification is to add each interaction term separately to the statistical model. When an interaction

Table 5.1. Results of a multilevel analysis of the effect of the intervention on total cholesterol

	Regression coefficient[1]	95% CI	p-value
'Crude'	−0.075	−0.489 to 0.339	0.72
'Adjusted'[2]	−0.119	−0.346 to 0.108	0.30

[1]Regression coefficient indicates the difference between the intervention and the control group at the end of the intervention period, corrected for baseline cholesterol values.
[2]Adjusted for BMI, smoking, gender, and age.

term is statistically significant, it indicates that the effect of the intervention is different for the different values of the effect modifier. Because the interaction terms have less power, the 'significance' levels of interaction terms are usually set slightly higher than 0.05 (e.g. p-values < 0.10). Outputs 5.12(a–e)

Output 5.12a. Results of a multilevel analysis to estimate the effect of the cholesterol-lowering intervention, with a random intercept and a random slope for the intervention variable, including the baseline cholesterol level and the interaction between the baseline cholesterol level and the intervention variable

---

```
total cholesterol_ij ~ N(XB, Ω)
total cholesterol_ij = β_0ij cons + 0,356(0,073) total cholesterol base_ij +
                       β_2j intervention_ij + -0,104(0,106) intervention*tc
                       base_ij
```

$\beta_{0ij} = 3{,}737(0{,}488) + u_{0j} + e_{0ij}$
$\beta_{2j} = 0{,}589(0{,}698) + u_{2j}$

$\begin{bmatrix} u_{0j} \\ u_{2j} \end{bmatrix} \sim N(0, \Omega_u) : \Omega_u = \begin{bmatrix} 0{,}331(0{,}159) \\ -0{,}316(0{,}159) & 0{,}334(0{,}174) \end{bmatrix}$

$[e_{0ij}] \sim N(0, \Omega_e) : \Omega_e = [0{,}349(0{,}031)]$

$-2*loglikelihood(IGLS) = 527{,}417 (276 \text{ of } 276 \text{ cases in use})$

Output 5.12b. Results of a multilevel analysis to estimate the effect of the cholesterol-lowering intervention, with a random intercept and a random slope for the intervention variable, including age and the interaction between age and the intervention variable

---

```
total cholesterol_ij ~ N(XB, Ω)
total cholesterol_ij = β_0ij cons + 0,186(0,053) total cholesterol base_ij +
                       β_2j intervention_ij + 0,054(0,009) age_ij +
                       -0,017(0,014) intervention*age_ij
```

$\beta_{0ij} = 2{,}783(0{,}416) + u_{0j} + e_{0ij}$
$\beta_{2j} = 0{,}532(0{,}576) + u_{2j}$

$\begin{bmatrix} u_{0j} \\ u_{2j} \end{bmatrix} \sim N(0, \Omega_u) : \Omega_u = \begin{bmatrix} 0{,}288(0{,}139) \\ -0{,}132(0{,}081) & 0{,}086(0{,}061) \end{bmatrix}$

$[e_{0ij}] \sim N(0, \Omega_e) : \Omega_e = [0{,}303(0{,}027)]$

$-2*loglikelihood(IGLS) = 488{,}641 (276 \text{ of } 276 \text{ cases in use})$

Output 5.12c. Results of a multilevel analysis to estimate the effect of the cholesterol-lowering intervention, with a random intercept and a random slope for the intervention variable, including BMI and the interaction between BMI and the intervention variable

```
total cholesterol_ij ~ N(XB, Ω)
total cholesterol_ij = β_0ij cons + 0,310(0,050)total cholesterol base_ij +
                       β_2j intervention_ij + 0,043(0,009)bmi_ij +
                       -0,015(0,014)intervention*bmi_ij
β_0ij = 2,643(0,455) + u_0j + e_0ij
β_2j = 0,423(0,482) + u_2j

[u_0j]  ~ N(0, Ω_u) : Ω_u = | 0,255(0,124)                |
[u_2j]                      | -0,280(0,141)  0,327(0,169) |
[e_0ij] ~ N(0, Ω_e) : Ω_e = [0,322(0,028)]

-2*loglikelihood(IGLS) = 501,269(276 of 276 cases in use)
```

Output 5.12d. Results of a multilevel analysis to estimate the effect of the cholesterol-lowering intervention, with a random intercept and a random slope for the intervention variable, including smoking and the interaction between smoking and the intervention variable

```
total cholesterol_ij ~ N(XB, Ω)
total cholesterol_ij = β_0ij cons + 0,302(0,052)total cholesterol base_ij +
                       β_2j intervention_ij + -0,354(0,113)smoking_ij +
                       0,423(0,169)intervention*smoking_ij
β_0ij = 4,283(0,382) + u_0j + e_0ij
β_2j = -0,329(0,218) + u_2j

[u_0j]  ~ N(0, Ω_u) : Ω_u = | 0,302(0,145)                |
[u_2j]                      | -0,284(0,145)  0,297(0,157) |
[e_0ij] ~ N(0, Ω_e) : Ω_e = [0,339(0,030)]

-2*loglikelihood(IGLS) = 518,557(276 of 276 cases in use)
```

Output 5.12e. Results of a multilevel analysis to estimate the effect of the cholesterol-lowering intervention, with a random intercept and a random slope for the intervention variable, including gender and the interaction between gender and the intervention variable

```
total cholesterolᵢⱼ ~ N(XB, Ω)
total cholesterolᵢⱼ = β₀ᵢⱼcons + 0,318(0,054)total cholesterol baseᵢⱼ +
                      β₂ⱼinterventionᵢⱼ + -0,155(0,118)genderᵢⱼ +
                      0,175(0,172)intervention*genderᵢⱼ

β₀ᵢⱼ = 4,022(0,385) + u₀ⱼ + e₀ᵢⱼ
β₂ⱼ = -0,137(0,225) + u₂ⱼ
```

$$\begin{bmatrix} u_{0j} \\ u_{2j} \end{bmatrix} \sim N(0, \ \Omega_u) \ : \ \Omega_u = \begin{bmatrix} 0,377(0,180) & \\ -0,370(0,183) & 0,387(0,198) \end{bmatrix}$$

$$[e_{0ij}] \sim N(0, \ \Omega_e) \ : \ \Omega_e = [0,348(0,031)]$$

```
-2*loglikelihood(IGLS) = 526,492(276 of 276 cases in use)
```

show the results of the multilevel analysis with the separate interaction terms, and Table 5.2 summarises the results of these analyses.

From the p-values of the interaction terms reported in Table 5.2 it can be seen that there is only a 'significant' interaction between the intervention variable and smoking. So, the effect of the intervention is significantly different for smokers and non-smokers. The implication of this significant interaction is that the effects of the intervention should be reported separately for smokers and non-smokers. It has been mentioned before in the discussion about confounding that it is recommended to report the results of both a 'crude' analysis and a 'corrected' analysis. So, in this situation, with a significant interaction between the intervention and smoking, a 'crude' result and an 'adjusted' result should be reported for smokers and for non-smokers.

Table 5.2. p-values belonging to different interaction terms to evaluate potential effect modification

	p-value
Intervention * baseline total cholesterol	0.592
Intervention * age	0.226
Intervention * BMI	0.285
Intervention * smoking	0.012
Intervention * gender	0.308

Both can be obtained by performing stratified analyses for smokers and non-smokers, but it is more elegant to use the analysis with the interaction term. Because non-smokers are coded as zero, the intervention effect, the 95% CI and the p-value for non-smokers can be obtained from the first analysis (the results of the 'crude' analysis were reported in Output 5.12d). The intervention effect (and 95% CI and p-value) for smokers can be obtained by first recoding the smoking variable (coding the smokers as zero). Then a 'new' interaction term has to be calculated (with the recoded smoking variable) and the data must be reanalysed. Outputs 5.13(a–d) show the results of these analyses, and Table 5.3 summarises the results.

From the results that are summarised in Table 5.3 it can be seen that there is a highly significant intervention effect for non-smokers, and that this effect is only significant when a correction has been made for age, BMI, and gender. Apparently, for smokers the intervention does not work. In fact, the positive regression coefficient observed for smokers indicates that, given a certain baseline value of total cholesterol, the intervention group has higher cholesterol values at follow-up, compared to the control group. It should be noted that in the present analysis a significant interaction was found for a dichotomous variable (i.e. smoking). For the different groups of the dichotomous variable (i.e. smokers and non-smokers), separate results can be reported. When a significant interaction is found with a continuous variable (e.g. age or

Output 5.13a. Results of a multilevel analysis to estimate the effect of the cholesterol-lowering intervention, with a random intercept and a random slope for the intervention variable, including smoking and the interaction between smoking and the intervention variable

$$\text{total cholesterol}_{ij} \sim N(XB, \ \Omega)$$

$$\text{total cholesterol}_{ij} = \beta_{0ij}\text{cons} + 0,302(0,052)\text{total cholesterol base}_{ij} +$$
$$\beta_{2j}\text{intervention}_{ij} + -0,354(0,113)\text{smoking}_{ij} +$$
$$0,423(0,169)\text{intervention*smoking}_{ij}$$

$$\beta_{0ij} = 4,283(0,382) + u_{0j} + e_{0ij}$$
$$\beta_{2j} = -0,329(0,218) + u_{2j}$$

$$\begin{bmatrix} u_{0j} \\ u_{2j} \end{bmatrix} \sim N(0, \ \Omega_u) \ : \ \Omega_u = \begin{bmatrix} 0,302(0,145) \\ -0,284(0,145) & 0,297(0,157) \end{bmatrix}$$

$$[e_{0ij}] \sim N(0, \ \Omega_e) \ : \ \Omega_e = [0,339(0,030)]$$

$$-2*loglikelihood(IGLS) = 518,557(276 \text{ of } 276 \text{ cases in use})$$

Output 5.13b. Results of a multilevel analysis to estimate the effect of the cholesterol-lowering intervention, with a random intercept and a random slope for the intervention variable, including smoking and the interaction between smoking and the intervention variable, corrected for age, BMI, and gender

```
total cholesterol_ij ~ N(XB, Ω)
total cholesterol_ij = β_0ijcons + 0,224(0,050)total cholesterol base_ij +
                       β_2jintervention_ij + 0,070(0,126)smoking_ij +
                       0,507(0,148)intervention*smoking_ij +
                       0,047(0,007)age_ij + 0,041(0,011)bmi_ij +
                       -0,126(0,114)gender_ij
β_0ij = 1,496(0,492) + u_0j + e_0ij
β_2j = -0,433(0,126) + u_2j
```

$$\begin{bmatrix} u_{0j} \\ u_{2j} \end{bmatrix} \sim N(0, \ \Omega_u) \ : \ \Omega_u = \begin{bmatrix} 0,202(0,099) \\ -0,056(0,046) & 0,024(0,030) \end{bmatrix}$$

$$[e_{0ij}] \sim N(0, \ \Omega_e) \ : \ \Omega_e = [0,275(0,024)]$$

```
-2*loglikelihood(IGLS) = 457,408(276 of 276 cases in use)
```

Output 5.13c. Results of a multilevel analysis to estimate the effect of the cholesterol-lowering intervention, with a random intercept and a random slope for the intervention variable, including smoking (recoded) and the interaction between smoking (recoded) and the intervention variable

```
total cholesterol_ij ~ N(XB, Ω)
total cholesterol_ij = β_0ijcons + 0,302(0,052)total cholesterol base_ij +
                       β_2jintervention_ij + 0,354(0,113)smoking_recode_ij +
                       -0,424(0,169)intervention*smoking_recode_ij
β_0ij = 3,933(0,372) + u_0j + e_0ij
β_2j = 0,095(0,197) + u_2j
```

$$\begin{bmatrix} u_{0j} \\ u_{2j} \end{bmatrix} \sim N(0, \ \Omega_u) \ : \ \Omega_u = \begin{bmatrix} 0,303(0,147) \\ -0,283(0,145) & 0,296(0,156) \end{bmatrix}$$

$$[e_{0ij}] \sim N(0, \ \Omega_e) \ : \ \Omega_e = [0,339(0,030)]$$

```
-2*loglikelihood(IGLS) = 518,555(276 of 276 cases in use)
```

Output 5.13d. Results of a multilevel analysis to estimate the effect of the cholesterol-lowering intervention, with a random intercept and a random slope for the intervention variable, including smoking (recoded) and the interaction between smoking (recoded) and the intervention variable, corrected for age, BMI, and gender

```
total cholesterol_ij ~ N(XB, Ω)
total cholesterol_ij = β_0ij cons + 0,224(0,050)total cholesterol base_ij +
                       β_2j intervention_ij + -0,070(0,126)smoking_recode_ij +
                       -0,507(0,148)intervention*smoking_recode_ij +
                       0,047(0,007)age_ij + 0,041(0,011)bmi_ij +
                       -0,126(0,114)gender_ij
β_0ij = 1,566(0,428) + u_0j + e_0ij
β_2j = 0,074(0,103) + u_2j

[u_0j]   ~ N(0, Ω_u) :  Ω_u = [ 0,202(0,099)                ]
[u_2j]                        [-0,056(0,046)  0,024(0,030) ]
[e_0ij] ~ N(0, Ω_e) :  Ω_e = [0,275(0,024)]

-2*loglikelihood(IGLS) = 457,407(276 of 276 cases in use)
```

BMI), the situation is slightly more complicated. There are basically two possibilities that are often used in this situation. The first possibility is to create two or more groups for the continuous variable and to estimate separate intervention effects for the different groups. However, the disadvantage of this method is that grouping a continuous variable not only leads to a loss of information, but it basically leads to a different variable. Another possibility is to report the 'average' intervention effect that can be obtained from an analysis

Table 5.3. Regression coefficients, 95% CI and p-values for the effect of a cholesterol-lowering intervention for smokers and non-smokers. Both 'crude' and 'adjusted'[1] results are presented

	Regression coefficient	95% CI	p-value
Non-smokers			
'Crude'	−0.329	−0.76 to 0.10	0.131
'Adjusted'[1]	−0.433	−0.68 to −0.19	<0.01
Smokers			
'Crude'	0.095	−0.29 to 0.48	0.631
'Adjusted'[1]	0.074	−0.13 to 0.28	0.472

[1]Adjusted for age, BMI, and gender.

without the interaction term, and report that a significant interaction was found with a particular continuous variable. Furthermore, it should be mentioned that this interaction has to interpreted in such a way that the intervention effect is stronger or weaker when the value of the continuous effect modifier is higher. Whether the effect is stronger or weaker depends on the sign of the regression coefficient for the intervention variable and the sign of the regression coefficient of the interaction term.

5.3.3   Prediction or prognostic models

The general idea underlying the construction of a prediction or prognostic model is that, given a certain set of independent variables, the best and most simple model (i.e. combination of independent variables) is constructed to predict the outcome variable of interest. In 'standard' regression analysis, prediction or prognostic models can be constructed manually, or automatically in the computer software. In general, there are two strategies that can be followed, a forward selection procedure or a backward selection procedure. With a forward selection procedure, the construction procedure starts by adding the independent variable that is most strongly associated with the outcome variable. This 'model' is then extended with the second best 'predictor', with the third best 'predictor', and so on, until a predefined end-point is reached. This endpoint can be that all variables included in the model must have a significant association with the outcome, but sometimes the cut-off value is somewhat higher (e.g. all variables with p-values < 0.10 are allowed in the model). With a backward selection procedure, the starting point is a model with all possible predictor variables. The modelling procedure starts by removing the independent variable that is least strongly associated with the outcome variable, and carries on removing these variables until it ends when a certain predefined end-point is reached. The automatic forward and backward selection procedures are not available in the MLwiN software, so all modelling must be done by hand. However, not only the significance of the independent variables is important, but also the random part of that relationship can be of importance. There are a few ways in which to construct a prediction or prognostic model, and unfortunately different modelling strategies do not always produce the same results. In the literature it is sometimes argued that in multilevel analysis, a backward strategy is preferred, and that one should start the modelling procedure with a 'full' model. A 'full' model is then defined as a model with not only all independent variables, but also all possible random variance components. This is theoretically probably the best approach that can be followed, but in practice it is not possible unless there is a very large study population. In most situations the coefficients of such a 'full' model can not be estimated, and therefore an alternative approach must be followed. In the next part of this chapter, an example will be given of an alternative strategy that can be followed to construct a prediction or prognostic model. It should be realised that this is just one of the possibilities; there are, of course, many more strategies available. In the example, total cholesterol is the outcome variable of interest, and the independent variables are age, gender, BMI, smoking, alcohol consumption and physical activity. Smoking is a dichotomous variable, while alcohol consumption and physical activity are categorised into three groups. For alcohol consumption, the first group consists of the non-drinkers and the second and third groups are divided by the median of the amount of alcohol consumed. Physical activity was divided into tertiles. Output 5.14 shows the descriptive information regarding the dataset used in this example.

Output 5.14. Descriptive information regarding the example dataset used to illustrate the construction of a prediction or prognostic model

| 1 | total cholester(| | | Refresh | Categories | Help | |

	Name	n	missing	min	max	
1	total cholesterol	441	0	3,9	8,86	
2	medical doctor	441	0	1	12	
3	age	441	0	44	86	
4	bmi	441	0	20,2	44,05	
5	physical activity	441	0	1	3	
6	smoking	441	0	0	1	
7	gender	441	0	0	1	
8	alcohol consumption	441	0	0	2	
9	activity dummy 1	441	0	0	1	
10	activity dummy 2	441	0	0	1	
11	alcohol dummy 1	441	0	0	1	
12	alcohol dummy 2	441	0	0	1	
13	id	441	0	1	441	
14	cons	441	0	1	1	

From Output 5.14 it can be seen that alcohol consumption and physical activity are represented by dummy variables. For both variables the lowest category is used as a reference category.

One of the possible modelling strategies starts with adding all potential predictor variables to the model. The next step is to evaluate whether or not a random intercept must be allowed. If a random intercept is necessary, the full model with a random intercept is the 'new' starting point. In this full model, for each of the predictor variables the importance must be evaluated for the situation with and the situation without a random slope for that particular variable. When this has been done for all predictor variables in the model, the variable with the lowest p-value can be deleted. Step by step this procedure must be repeated until a certain predefined end-point is reached. Again, this end-point is usually reached when all independent variables in the model are significant, but sometimes a somewhat less restrictive end-point is used. When the procedure described above has been followed in the example dataset, the model as shown in Output 5.15 is found to be the best and most simple model to predict total cholesterol.

From Output 5.15 it can be seen that the best and most simple model to predict total cholesterol consists of age, BMI, and smoking. It can further be seen that for both age and smoking a random slope is considered. It is

Output 5.15. Results of a multilevel model to predict total cholesterol values, allowing both a random intercept and random slopes

$$\text{total cholesterol}_{ij} \sim N(XB, \ \Omega)$$
$$\text{total cholesterol}_{ij} = \beta_{0ij}\text{cons} + \beta_{1j}\text{age}_{ij} + 0,069144\,(0,008983)\text{bmi}_{ij} +$$
$$\beta_{3j}\text{smoking}_{ij}$$

$\beta_{0ij} = 0,733683\,(0,485653) + u_{0j} + e_{0ij}$
$\beta_{1j} = 0,044302\,(0,005119) + u_{1j}$
$\beta_{3j} = 0,486475\,(0,126070) + u_{3j}$

$$\begin{bmatrix} u_{0j} \\ u_{1j} \\ u_{3j} \end{bmatrix} \sim N(0, \ \Omega_u) : \Omega_u = \begin{bmatrix} 1,327741(0,727363) & & \\ -0,013988(0,009002) & 0,000198(0,000125) & \\ -0,151959(0,145022) & 0,000960(0,001788) & 0,063220(0,046632) \end{bmatrix}$$

$[e_{0ij}] \sim N(0, \ \Omega_e) : \Omega_e = [0,274169(0,019205)]$

$-2*\text{loglikelihood}(IGLS) = 744,807100\,(441 \text{ of } 441 \text{ cases in use})$

interesting to compare the results of this modelling procedure with the results of other strategies. When the multilevel structure is ignored, and therefore a 'naive' prediction model is constructed, the results are remarkably different (see Output 5.16), not with regard to the variables that are present in the model, but in terms of the magnitudes of the regression coefficients and corresponding standard errors.

Output 5.16. Results of a 'naive' model to predict total cholesterol values

```
total cholesterolᵢⱼ ~ N(XB, Ω)
total cholesterolᵢⱼ = β₀ᵢcons + 0,044850(0,003744)ageᵢⱼ +
                       0,098977(0,010651)bmiᵢⱼ +
                       0,351121(0,124843)smokingᵢⱼ
β₀ᵢ = -0,126048(0,431681) + e₀ᵢⱼ

[e₀ᵢⱼ] ~ N(0, Ωₑ) : Ωₑ = [0,515193(0,034695)]

-2*loglikelihood(IGLS) = 959,026700(441 of 441 cases in use)
```

A slightly less 'naive' approach is a modelling strategy in which a random intercept is allowed, but random slopes are not allowed. Output 5.17 shows the results of the final model derived from this modelling strategy.

Output 5.17. Results of a multilevel model to predict total cholesterol values, allowing only a random intercept

```
total cholesterolᵢⱼ ~ N(XB, Ω)
total cholesterolᵢⱼ = β₀ᵢⱼcons + 0,050660(0,003408)ageᵢⱼ +
                       0,053807(0,010585)bmiᵢⱼ + 0,487466(0,161520)smokingᵢⱼ +
                       -0,010429(0,064071)activity dummy 1ᵢⱼ +
                       -0,261227(0,083753)activity dummy 2ᵢⱼ +
                       0,255799(0,143794)alcohol dummy 1ᵢⱼ +
                       0,165505(0,084851)alcohol dummy 2ᵢⱼ
β₀ᵢⱼ = 0,739135(0,435395) + u₀ⱼ + e₀ᵢⱼ

[u₀ⱼ] ~ N(0, Ωᵤ) : Ωᵤ = [0,299533(0,125407)]

[e₀ᵢⱼ] ~ N(0, Ωₑ) : Ωₑ = [0,284631(0,019435)]

-2*loglikelihood(IGLS) = 741,522300(441 of 441 cases in use)
```

Table 5.4. Regression coefficients and standard errors (between brackets) derived from different models in order to predict total cholesterol values

	'Naive'	Only random intercept	Random intercept and random slopes
Age	0.045 (0.004)	0.051 (0.003)	0.044 (0.005)
BMI	0.099 (0.011)	0.054 (0.011)	0.069 (0.009)
Smoking	0.351 (0.124)	0.487 (0.162)	0.486 (0.126)
Gender			
Activity[1]			
Moderate	−0.010 (0.064)		
High	−0.261 (0.084)		
Alcohol[2]			
Moderate	0.256 (0.144)		
Heavy	0.166 (0.085)		

[1]Physical activity was divided into tertiles and the lowest tertile was used as reference category.
[2]No alcohol consumption was used as reference category; moderate and heavy alcohol consumers are divided by the median of the amount of alcohol consumed.

From Output 5.17 it can be seen that a totally different model has been constructed with this strategy. In addition to age, BMI, and smoking, physical activity and alcohol consumption are also present in the final model. The last strategy (i.e. with only a random intercept) looks a bit artificial, but it is not. In some software packages, only a random intercept can be allowed, and therefore the final model that has been shown in Output 5.17 will be the final prediction or prognostic model. To summarise the results of the different modelling procedures that are described in this section, Table 5.4 shows the regression coefficients and standard errors of the variables included in the 'final' models. It should (again) be realised that the three modelling strategies described in this section are examples of possible modelling strategies, and that there are other (maybe even better) modelling strategies available. Important, however, is the fact that the result of a final prediction or prognostic model (highly) depends on the modelling strategy that is chosen.

In the three strategies to construct a prediction or prognostic model, we did not include any interaction terms. Although theoretically interaction terms can be part of the final prediction or prognostic model, in practice this is hardly ever done. In most practical situations, it is decided a priori (e.g. based on biological plausibility) that stratified prediction or prognostic models are going to be constructed. For instance, it can be decided (a priori) that separate prediction or prognostic models are going to be constructed for males and females.

5.4 Comments

In the examples in this chapter, a continuous outcome variable was used. However, dealing with confounding and effect modification as well as the construction of association and prediction or prognostic models is exactly the same for dichotomous, categorical or 'count' outcome variables.

6

Multilevel analysis in longitudinal studies

6.1 Introduction

In the earlier chapters it has been explained that multilevel analysis is suitable for the analysis of correlated data. We have seen examples in which observations of patients were correlated because they 'belong' to the same medical doctor, i.e. the observations of patients were clustered within medical doctors. The fact that observations are correlated is probably most pronounced in longitudinal studies in which repeated observations are made within one subject or patient. It is obvious that these observations are (usually) highly correlated. Therefore, the whole theory of multilevel analysis, as described in the earlier chapters, can also be applied to longitudinal data. With longitudinal data, the repeated observations are clustered within the subject or patient (see Figure 6.1).

Figure 6.1 illustrates a two-level structure, i.e. the observations are the lower level, while the patient is the higher level. This is different from all the examples that have been described before, in which the patients were the lower level. It is of course also possible that the patients are clustered within medical doctors, as was also the situation in the earlier chapters. This is referred to as a three-level structure, i.e. the observations are clustered within the patients and the patients are clustered within the medical doctors (see Figure 6.2).

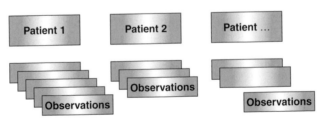

Figure 6.1. Two-level longitudinal multilevel structure; observations are clustered within patients.

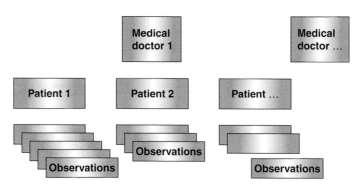

Figure 6.2. Three-level longitudinal multilevel structure; observations are clustered within patients and patients are clustered with medical doctors.

6.2 Longitudinal studies

Longitudinal studies are characterised by the fact that the outcome variable is repeatedly measured over time. Table 6.1 shows an example of a typical longitudinal dataset.

From Table 6.1 it can be seen that all patients are measured four times, and that the outcome variable is continuous. There are two independent variables, one time-dependent continuous variable and another time-independent dichotomous variable. Furthermore, there is a variable called *time* that consists of the 'observation number' for each patient. It should be noted that this dataset has a so-called 'long' data structure, which means that there is one record for each observation. In contrast with the 'long' data structure, there is also a so-called 'broad' data structure, in which there is one record for each patient (the broad data structure is the standard data structure used, for instance, in SPSS, and repeated observations are usually referred to as *y1*, *y2*, *y3*, etc.). However, a 'long' data structure is necessary for longitudinal data analysis.

Suppose, we are interested in the (longitudinal) relationship between the outcome variable Y and the time-dependent determinant X_1. Ignoring the fact that the observations are clustered within the patients (i.e. ignoring the multilevel structure of the data), 'standard' linear regression analysis can be applied (Equation (6.1)):

$$Y = \beta_0 + \beta_1 X_1 + \varepsilon \tag{6.1}$$

where Y = outcome variable; β_0 = intercept; β_1 = regression coefficient for X_1; X_1 = time-dependent independent variable; and ε = error/residual.

Table 6.1. Hypothetical example of a typical longitudinal dataset

Patient	Outcome variable (Y)	Time-dependent determinant (X_1)	Time-independent determinant (X_2)	Time
1	3.5	2.4	1	1
1	3.7	4.3	1	2
1	4.2	4.5	1	3
1	4.5	5.1	1	4
2	1.4	2.8	0	1
2	1.6	2.9	0	2
2	1.7	3.0	0	3
2	1.8	2.7	0	4
.				
.				
.				
N	5.6	5.0	0	1
N	5.6	5.1	0	2
N	5.7	7.5	0	3
N	5.8	6.3	0	4

There are probably very few researchers who would perform a 'standard' linear regression analysis on longitudinal data. Everybody is aware of the fact that something different should be done because the observations are clustered within one patient. To cope with this (comparable to the situation in which observations of patients are clustered within medical doctors), a correction can be made for 'patient' (Equation (6.2)):

$$Y = \beta_0 + \beta_1 X_1 + \beta_2 \text{pat} + \varepsilon \tag{6.2}$$

where β_2 = regression coefficient for the 'patient' variable.

However, performing a linear regression analysis according to Equation (6.2) is impossible, because the 'patient' variable is not a continuous or dichotomous variable. It is a categorical (i.e. nominal) variable that must be represented by dummy variables (Equation (6.3)):

$$Y = \beta_0 + \beta_1 X_1 + \beta_2 \text{pat}_1 + \beta_3 \text{pat}_2 + \cdots \beta_n \text{pat}_{n-1} + \varepsilon \tag{6.3}$$

where β_2 = regression coefficient for the dummy variable representing the first patient; pat_1 = dummy variable representing the first patient; β_3 = regression coefficient for the dummy variable representing the second patient; $pat_2 =$ dummy variable representing the second patient; $pat_{n-1} =$ dummy variable representing the $(n - 1)$th patient, etc.; and $n =$ number of patients.

In fact, a correction for 'patient' means that different intercepts are estimated for each patient (see Figure 6.3).

As a typical longitudinal study usually consists of a few repeated measurements of many patients, the number of dummy variables will be huge, compared to the total number of observations, and therefore it would be impossible to analyse the data in this way. To deal with this, again, multilevel analysis provides a very elegant solution, i.e. it is not the separate intercepts for each patient that are estimated, but the variance of those intercepts. So, instead of many regression coefficients for all dummy variables (representing each patient), only one variance parameter (i.e. a 'random intercept') is estimated. Of course, the assumption of this 'random intercept' is that the different intercepts are normally distributed (see also Sections 2.2 and 2.7).

In line with this, it can also be hypothesised that not only the intercepts differ between the patients, but also the relationship between Y and X_1. In 'standard' linear regression analysis this can be analysed by adding the interaction between X_1 and patient to the regression equation (Equation (6.4)):

$$Y = \beta_0 + \beta_1 X_1 + \beta_2 pat + \beta_3 pat \times X_1 + \varepsilon \tag{6.4}$$

where $\beta_3 =$ regression coefficient for the interaction between the 'patient' variable and the time-dependent determinant X_1.

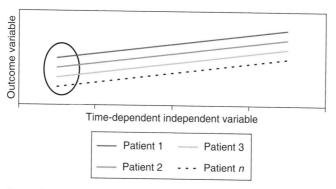

Figure 6.3. Illustration of a linear regression analysis of a time-dependent independent variable and a certain outcome variable with a different intercept for each patient.

Just as in the correction for the 'patient' variable, the interaction terms should also be represented by dummy variables (Equation (6.5)):

$$Y = \beta_0 + \beta_1 X_1 + \beta_2 \text{pat}_1 + \beta_3 \text{pat}_2 + \cdots + \beta_n \text{pat}_{n-1}$$
$$+ \beta_{n+1} \text{pat}_1 \times X_1 + \beta_{n+2} \text{pat}_2 \times X_1 + \cdots + \beta_{2n-1} \text{pat}_{n-1} + \varepsilon \qquad (6.5)$$

where β_{n+1} = regression coefficient for the interaction between the dummy variable representing the first patient and X_1; β_{n+2} = regression coefficient for the interaction between the dummy variable representing the second patient and X_1; β_{2n-1} = regression coefficient for the interaction between the dummy variable representing the $(n-1)$th patient and X_1.

Just as in the correction for the 'patient' variable, for the interaction between the 'patient' variable and the time-dependent determinant X_1, a large number of regression coefficients must also be estimated. Given the nature of most longitudinal studies (i.e. a few repeated measurements of many patients), this would also be impossible. Again, an elegant solution for this problem is multilevel analysis, in which not all the regression coefficients for each patient are estimated separately, but in which the variance of the regression coefficients is estimated (see Figure 6.4). Just as for the random intercepts, a normal distribution is also assumed for the random slopes!

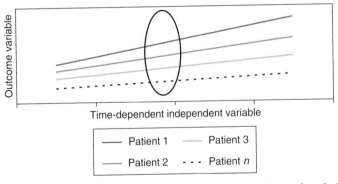

Figure 6.4. Illustration of a linear regression analysis of a time-dependent independent variable and a certain outcome variable with a different intercept and a different slope for each patient.

6.3 Example

To illustrate the use of multilevel analysis for longitudinal data, an observational longitudinal study in which four measurements are performed on 147
patients is used as an example. The question to be answered is whether
lifestyle influences health. Output 6.1 shows descriptive information regarding the dataset.

Output 6.1. Descriptive information regarding the example longitudinal
dataset

	Name	n	missing	min	max
1	id	588	0	1	147
2	health indicator	588	0	2,4	6,4
3	lifestyle indicator	588	0	1,57	9,05
4	time	588	0	1	4
5	cons	588	0	1	1

(window controls: 1 id   Refresh   Categories   Help)

From Output 6.1 it can be seen that 588 observations are performed (i.e.
four measurements of 147 patients). The second column shows the values for
the health indicator (i.e. the outcome variable) and the third column shows
the values for the lifestyle indicator (i.e. the time-dependent independent
variable). It can be seen that there are no missing data, although this would
not be a problem for the estimation of the regression coefficients (see Section
6.6.3). The fourth column gives the *time* variable, which represents the
'observation number' for each patient, and ranges from 1 to 4. The last column of the dataset gives the *cons* variable, which (again) consists only of ones
and is necessary to estimate an intercept in multilevel regression analysis.

Output 6.2 shows the results of a 'naive' analysis in which all observations
are considered to be independent. Again, it is rather strange to analyse
the data in this way, but it is explained in this section just for educational

purposes. The results will be compared with the results of a 'proper' analysis in which it is taken into account that the repeated measurements of the same patient 'belong' to each other (i.e. that the repeated observations are clustered within patients).

Output 6.2. Results of a 'naive' longitudinal multilevel analysis of the relationship between health and lifestyle

```
health indicatorᵢⱼ ~ N(XB, Ω)
health indicatorᵢⱼ = β₀ᵢcons + 0,141(0,020)lifestyle indicatorᵢⱼ

β₀ᵢ = 3,808(0,073) + e₀ᵢⱼ

[e₀ᵢⱼ] ~ N(0, Ωₑ) : Ωₑ = [0,439(0,026)]

-2*loglikelihood(IGLS) = 1184,665(588 of 588 cases in use)
```

From Output 6.2 it can be seen that there is a highly significant association between lifestyle and health. The Wald statistic for this association is $(0.141/0.020)^2 = 49.7$, which follows a Chi-square distribution with one degree of freedom and is highly significant. It should be noted that the subscript i of the variables in the regression equation represents the observation, while the subscript j represents the patient. This is because the observations are clustered within the patients and the lowest level is always noted as i, while the second level is always noted as j.

To perform a 'real' longitudinal analysis, a random intercept is added to the analysis. So, a correction is made for 'patient', or, in other words, in this analysis it is taken into account that repeated observations are made within the same patient. Output 6.3 shows the results of this analysis.

Two important aspects should be noted in Output 6.3. First of all, it can be seen that the magnitude of the association between lifestyle and health has changed dramatically. When a correction is made for 'patient' (i.e. when a random intercept is allowed), the magnitude of the regression coefficient for lifestyle decreased from 0.141 to 0.070, while the standard error remained more or less the same. When the Wald test is applied in this situation (i.e. $[0.070/0.023]^2 = 9.25$), the association is still highly significant.

Output 6.3. Results of a linear longitudinal multilevel analysis of the relationship between health and lifestyle with a random intercept

```
health indicator_ij ~ N(XB, Ω)
health indicator_ij = β_0ijcons + 0,070(0,023)lifestyle indicator_ij
β_0ij = 4,054(0,094) + u_0j + e_0ij

[u_0j] ~ N(0, Ω_u)  :  Ω_u = [0,321(0,041)]
[e_0ij] ~ N(0, Ω_e)  :  Ω_e = [0,128(0,009)]

-2*loglikelihood(IGLS) = 812,006(588 of 588 cases in use)
```

The second aspect that should be noted is the amount of variance that is 'explained' by correction for the patient. The intraclass correlation coefficient (ICC), which is an indicator of the dependency of the repeated observations within the patients can be estimated by dividing the between-patient variance (i.e. 0.321) by the total variance (i.e. 0.321 + 0.128). The ICC in this example is 0.71. This relatively high ICC is, however, not uncommon in longitudinal studies. In general, the ICC observed in longitudinal multilevel analysis (representing the correlation of repeated observations within patients) is much higher than the ICC observed in cross-sectional multilevel analysis.

In order to evaluate whether or not it is necessary to allow a random intercept, the likelihood ratio test can be applied (which is of course highly significant), although in longitudinal studies it is a conceptual necessity to allow the intercepts for each patient to be different; in fact that is basically the whole idea of a longitudinal study.

The second step in the multilevel modelling process is the addition of a random slope (i.e. adding the interaction between lifestyle and 'patient' to the model). Output 6.4 shows the result of this analysis.

From the fourth line of Output 6.4 it can be seen that a random slope for health is added to the analysis. The regression coefficient for the lifestyle indicator is extended with a variance component (i.e. u_{1j}). The magnitude of this variance component (i.e. 0.010) is shown in the variance/covariance matrix in the fifth and sixth line of the output. From this matrix it can also be seen that the covariance between the random intercept and the random

Output 6.4. Results of a linear longitudinal multilevel analysis of the relationship between health and lifestyle with both a random intercept and a random slope for lifestyle

```
health indicator_ij ~ N(XB, Ω)
health indicator_ij = β_0ij cons + β_1j lifestyle indicator_ij
β_0ij = 4,046(0,102) + u_0j + e_0ij
β_1j = 0,072(0,025) + u_1j
```

$$\begin{bmatrix} u_{0j} \\ u_{1j} \end{bmatrix} \sim N(0, \ \Omega_u) : \Omega_u = \begin{bmatrix} 0,511(0,170) \\ -0,046(0,039) \ 0,010(0,009) \end{bmatrix}$$

```
[e_0ij] ~ N(0, Ω_e)  : Ω_e = [0,124(0,009)]
```

```
-2*loglikelihood(IGLS) = 810,237(588 of 588 cases in use)
```

slope has a negative sign. This indicates that for patients with a relatively high intercept the association between health and lifestyle is weaker. It has been mentioned before that allowing a random intercept is a conceptual necessity, but this is not the case for allowing a random slope. Therefore, a likelihood ratio test should be applied to evaluate whether or not a random slope should be considered. For the likelihood ratio test, the −2 log likelihood of the model with only a random intercept (see Output 6.3) must be compared to the −2 log likelihood of the model with both a random intercept and a random slope (see Output 6.4). This difference is 812.006 − 810.237 = 1.769, and follows a Chi-square distribution with two degrees of freedom (two degrees of freedom, because both the random slope and the covariance between the random intercept and random slope are estimated), which has a (two-sided) p-value of 0.184, i.e. not significant. Whether a one- or two-sided p-value should be used in this situation has already been discussed in Section 2.2, but has no influence on the final conclusion, which is that it is not necessary to allow the regression coefficients for the lifestyle indicator to be random. So, the final result of this analysis is that there is a positive association between lifestyle and health, and the magnitude of that association is 0.070, with a 95% confidence interval (CI) ranging from 0.025 to 0.115 and a p-value < 0.001. The interpretation of the regression coefficient is rather complicated, and is basically twofold, a between-patient interpretation, and a within-patient interpretation. The between-patient interpretation is comparable with the 'normal' interpretation of a regression coefficient. When two patients differ one unit in the lifestyle indicator, they differ 0.070 units in the health indicator. The within-patient interpretation is typical for a longitudinal study. When health increases with one unit over a particular time-period within a patient, this change is accompanied by an increase of 0.070 units in the health of that patient. Of course, the total regression coefficient of 0.070 is partly between patients and partly within patients. It is possible to discriminate between the two interpretations by performing a so-called autoregressive longitudinal analysis. For a detailed discussion about this 'pooled' interpretation and autoregressive longitudinal analysis, reference is made to Twisk (2003).

In the example the longitudinal relationship with a continuous outcome variable was analysed. It should be noted that multilevel analysis can also be used to analyse longitudinal relationships with dichotomous and categorical outcome variables.

6.4 Growth curves

In epidemiological and medical longitudinal studies, multilevel analysis is probably most often applied for the construction of growth curves (see, for instance, Plewis, 1996; Plewis, 2000; Boyle and Willms, 2001; Beunen et al., 2002; Baxter-Jones et al., 2003; Heo et al., 2003; Hernández-Lloreda et al., 2003; Thompson et al., 2003). Growth curves are used to describe the development over time of a particular outcome variable. This specific topic will be explained with the same example that was used in Section 6.3. So, the dataset is the same as in Output 6.1. In the example dataset four measurements are made of each patient, so basically a third-degree polynomial is the highest order growth curve that can be modelled. Let us first start with a linear development over time. Output 6.5 shows the result of an analysis with only *time* as an independent variable, and with a random intercept. Again, a random intercept is a conceptual necessity in longitudinal studies, so it is basically not necessary to evaluate this by performing a likelihood ratio test. It is, furthermore, important to realise that in growth curve analysis the lowest level (i.e. *observation* or *time*) is also the only (or most important) independent variable.

Output 6.5. Results of a linear multilevel 'growth curve' analysis for health, with a random intercept

```
health indicator_ij ~ N(XB, Ω)
health indicator_ij = β_0ij cons + -0,084(0,013)time_ij
β_0ij = 4,510(0,060) + u_0j + e_0ij

[u_0j] ~ N(0, Ω_u)  :  Ω_u = [0,354(0,045)]
[e_0ij] ~ N(0, Ω_e)  :  Ω_e = [0,115(0,008)]

-2*loglikelihood(IGLS) = 777,822(588 of 588 cases in use)
```

From Output 6.5 it can be seen that health is decreasing over time. The regression coefficient for *time* is −0.084, so for each measurement health decreases with 0.084 points. Whether or not this linear decrease over time is significant, can be evaluated from the Wald statistic $(-0.084/0.013)^2 = 41.74$, which is Chi-square distributed with one degree of freedom, i.e. highly significant. When the result of this analysis is compared to a 'naive' analysis in which the dependency of the observations is ignored (see Output 6.6), it can be seen that the regression coefficient for *time* is exactly the same, but that the standard error in the 'corrected' analysis is lower than in the 'naive' analysis. This is typical for growth curve analysis, or, in general, this is typical for longitudinal studies when the independent variable is time dependent. In these situations the standard error of the regression coefficient decreases, when a random intercept is allowed (Twisk, 2003). This is in contrast with cross-sectional studies (see Chapter 3) and longitudinal studies in which a time-independent independent variable is analysed.

Output 6.6. Results of a 'naive' linear multilevel 'growth curve' analysis for health

```
health indicator_ij ~ N(XB, Ω)
health indicator_ij = β_0i cons + -0,084(0,025)time_ij
β_0i = 4,509(0,069) + e_0ij

[e_0ij] ~ N(0, Ω_e)  :  Ω_e = [0,469(0,027)]

-2*loglikelihood(IGLS) = 1223,576(588 of 588 cases in use)
```

The next step in the linear growth curve analysis can be the extension of the model with a random slope for *time*. Output 6.7 shows the result of this analysis.

Output 6.7. Results of a linear multilevel 'growth curve' analysis for health, with both a random intercept and a random slope

```
health indicator_ij ~ N(XB, Ω)
health indicator_ij = β_0ij cons + β_1j time_ij
β_0ij = 4,510(0,060) + u_0j + e_0ij
β_1j = -0,084(0,015) + u_1j
```

$$\begin{bmatrix} u_{0j} \\ u_{1j} \end{bmatrix} \sim N(0, \ \Omega_u) : \Omega_u = \begin{bmatrix} 0{,}391(0{,}062) & \\ -0{,}026(0{,}013) & 0{,}016(0{,}004) \end{bmatrix}$$

```
[e_0ij] ~ N(0, Ω_e) : Ω_e = [0,089(0,007)]

-2*loglikelihood(IGLS) = 754,374(588 of 588 cases in use)
```

The extension of the model with a random slope for *time* (indicated by u_{1j}) has resulted in a decrease in the −2 log likelihood. In the model without a random slope, the −2 log likelihood was 777.822 (see Output 6.5), while the −2 log likelihood in the model with a random slope with time is 754.374. The likelihood ratio test therefore gives a value of 23.448, which follows a Chi-square distribution with two degrees of freedom, and is highly significant. Again, there are two degrees of freedom, because not only the random slope for *time* is estimated, but also the covariance between the random intercept and the random slope. From the negative sign of this covariance it can be interpreted that for patients with a high intercept the decrease over time is greater than for patients with a relatively low intercept.

Up to now, a linear development over time has been modelled. However, it is also possible that the development is better described by a second- or third-order polynomial with time. So, the next step in the analysis can be to extend the model with a *time²* variable. Output 6.8 shows the result of this analysis.

To evaluate whether or not a second-order polynomial should be used to describe the longitudinal development over time, the Wald statistic for *time²* can be calculated. In the present example this Wald statistic is $(0.005/0.012)^2 = 0.17$, which follows a Chi-square distribution with one degree of

Output 6.8. Results of a second-order multilevel 'growth curve' analysis for health, with a random intercept and a random slope for the linear component of time

```
health indicator_ij ~ N(XB, Ω)
health indicator_ij = β_0ij cons + β_1j time_ij + 0,005(0,012)time2_ij
β_0ij = 4,533(0,086) + u_0j + e_0ij
β_1j = -0,108(0,063) + u_1j
```

$$\begin{bmatrix} u_{0j} \\ u_{1j} \end{bmatrix} \sim N(0, \; \Omega_u) : \Omega_u = \begin{bmatrix} 0,392(0,062) & \\ -0,026(0,013) & 0,016(0,004) \end{bmatrix}$$

```
[e_0ij] ~ N(0, Ω_e)  : Ω_e = [0,089(0,007)]

-2*loglikelihood(IGLS) = 754,223(588 of 588 cases in use)
```

freedom, and the corresponding p-value is 0.680. This is not significant, so a second-order polynomial is not necessary. The same procedure can be followed for the evaluation of a possible third-order polynomial. Output 6.9 shows the results of an analysis in which *time*, *time²*, and *time³* are added as independent variables.

Output 6.9. Results of a third-order multilevel 'growth curve' analysis for health, with a random intercept and a random slope for the linear component of time

```
health indicator_ij ~ N(XB, Ω)
health indicator_ij = β_0ij cons + β_1j time_ij +
                      0,117(0,138)time2_ij +
                      -0,015(0,018)time3_ij
β_0ij = 4,691(0,210) + u_0j + e_0ij
β_1j = -0,358(0,312) + u_1j
```

$$\begin{bmatrix} u_{0j} \\ u_{1j} \end{bmatrix} \sim N(0, \; \Omega_u) : \Omega_u = \begin{bmatrix} 0,392(0,062) & \\ -0,026(0,013) & 0,016(0,004) \end{bmatrix}$$

```
[e_0ij] ~ N(0, Ω_e)  : Ω_e = [0,088(0,007)]

-2*loglikelihood(IGLS) = 753,553(588 of 588 cases in use)
```

Just like the Wald statistic for $time^2$, the Wald statistic for $time^3$ is also not statistically significant (i.e. $[-0.015/0.018]^2 = 0.69$; p-value $= 0.406$), so the conclusion of the two analyses is that the development over time for the health indicator is best described by a linear function, with both a random intercept and a random slope for $time$ (see Output 6.7). It should be noted that there are different ways to obtain this conclusion. Some authors suggest that you should always start with a model that is as big as possible (i.e. with all possible random variances), and then exclude variances as well as variables with a backward selection procedure (see also Section 5.3.3). However, constructing the growth curve in the way that is described in this section provides more insight into the data and more insight into the steps that are taken. Especially for researchers with (very) little experience in multilevel modelling, the procedure described here is (probably) recommendable.

In the example, only possible polynomial functions with time are illustrated. However, it also possible to model other functions with time, such as logistic, logarithmic, or exponential functions.

When discrete time points are used in a longitudinal study (as in the present example), $time$ can also be modelled as a categorical variable. In the example four measurements were made of each patient, so the categorical $time$ variable must be represented by three dummy variables. The regression coefficients belonging to each of these dummy variables indicate the difference between a certain time point and a reference point (which is usually the first (baseline) measurement). Output 6.10 shows the results of an analysis in which the development over time for the health indicator is modelled with three dummy variables for the categorical $time$ variable. The first measurement is used as a reference category, and in the analysis (only) a random intercept is allowed.

From Output 6.10 it can be seen that there are three dummy variables for time. The regression coefficient belonging to the first dummy variable represents the difference in the health indicator between the first and the second measurement. This difference is -0.112, with a standard error of 0.040. The corresponding p-value is again based on the Wald statistic (i.e. $[-0.112/0.040]^2 = 7.84$), which follows a Chi-square distribution with one degree of freedom ($p < 0.001$). The regression coefficient for the second dummy variable represents the difference in the health indicator between the first and the third measurement. This difference is -0.169, and the

Output 6.10. Results of a multilevel 'growth curve' analysis for health, with time treated as a categorical variable (i.e. represented by dummy variables), with a random intercept

```
health indicator_{ij} ~ N(XB, Ω)
health indicator_{ij} = β_{0ij}cons + -0,112(0,040)time dummy1_{ij} +
                        -0,169(0,040)time dummy2_{ij} +
                        -0,261(0,040)time dummy3_{ij}

β_{0ij} = 4,435(0,056) + u_{0j} + e_{0ij}

[u_{0j}] ~ N(0, Ω_u) : Ω_u = [0,354(0,045)]
[e_{0ij}] ~ N(0, Ω_e) : Ω_e = [0,115(0,008)]

-2*loglikelihood(IGLS) = 777,191(588 of 588 cases in use)
```

corresponding p-value is again based on the Wald statistic (i.e. $[-0.169/0.040]^2 = 17.85$), and is < 0.001. Finally, the regression coefficient belonging to the third dummy variable represents the difference between the first measurement and the fourth measurement. In the present example this difference is -0.261, which is also highly significant (i.e. $[-0.261/0.040]^2 = 42.58$; p-value < 0.001).

The next step in this analysis is an extension with random slopes for the three dummy variables. However, this analysis did not lead to a valid result. After some trial and error, a (final) model was obtained with a random intercept and only random slopes for the second and the third dummy variables. Output 6.11 shows the results of this analysis.

To evaluate whether or not the addition of random slopes for the second and the third dummy variable is necessary, the likelihood ratio test can be applied. To do so, the -2 log likelihood of the model with only a random intercept (i.e. 777.191; Output 6.10) must be compared to the -2 log likelihood of the model with the two random slopes (i.e. 753.661; Output 6.11). The difference between the two is 25.53, which follows a Chi-square distribution with five degrees of freedom (five degrees of freedom, because in addition to the two variances for the slopes, three covariances are also estimated). The corresponding p-value is < 0.001. So, in conclusion, the model with the random slopes for the second dummy variable (i.e. representing the

Output 6.11. Results of a multilevel 'growth curve' analysis for health, with time treated as a categorical variable (i.e. represented by dummy variables), with a random intercept and random slopes for the second and the third dummy variables for time

---

health indicator$_{ij}$ ~ N(XB, Ω)

health indicator$_{ij}$ = β_{0ij}cons + -0,112(0,038)time dummy1$_{ij}$ + β_{2j}time dummy2$_{ij}$ + β_{3j}time dummy3$_{ij}$

β_{0ij} = 4,435(0,055) + u_{0j} + e_{0ij}

β_{2j} = -0,169(0,041) + u_{2j}

β_{3j} = -0,261(0,042) + u_{3j}

$$\begin{bmatrix} u_{0j} \\ u_{2j} \\ u_{3j} \end{bmatrix} \sim N(0, \ \Omega_u) : \Omega_u = \begin{bmatrix} 0,337(0,046) \\ 0,010(0,024) & 0,029(0,029) \\ 0,001(0,025) & 0,068(0,020) & 0,041(0,030) \end{bmatrix}$$

$[e_{0ij}]$ ~ N(0, Ω_e) : Ω_e = [0,109(0,013)]

$-2*loglikelihood(IGLS)$ = 753,661(588 of 588 cases in use)

---

difference between the first and third measurement) and for the third dummy variable (i.e. representing the difference between the first and the fourth measurement) is 'better' than the model without the random slopes. So, the final growth curve should be based on the model, which is shown in Output 6.11. Based on these results the differences, 95% CIs and corresponding p-values must be obtained.

It should be noted that the procedure which treats the *time* variable as categorical is only possible when discrete time-points are considered. When the actual time is used for the construction of growth curves, a certain function over time must be assumed. An example of the construction of a growth curve using actual time is given in the next section.

6.4.1 An additional example

A nice example of growth curve modelling can be found in a study by Gerards et al. (2004, 2005). In this study, the longitudinal development of lung volumes in foetuses is analysed. All 49 foetuses were measured three to four times, but not at predefined time-points. They were measured at some time during the gestation period (i.e. somewhere between 17 and 35 weeks), and preferably there was an interval of 4 weeks between each measurement. So basically, this study is partly longitudinal (each foetus is measured three or four times), and partly cross-sectional (the gestation age range for the total population is larger than the gestation age range for each individual foetus). Table 6.2 shows part of the dataset and Output 6.12 gives descriptive information about this dataset.

Table 6.2. Part of the dataset used to create a growth curve for lung volume in foetuses

Patient	Lung volume (ml)	Weeks
1	9.06	18.0
1	24.33	22.6
1	49.03	26.0
1	64.83	30.0
2	9.03	18.0
2	16.41	22.0
2	14.21	26.0
2	64.37	30.0
⋮	⋮	⋮
⋮	⋮	⋮
52	11.36	20.9
52	29.44	25.0
52	41.83	29.0
52	69.34	33.7

Output 6.12. Descriptive information regarding the additional example of the 'growth curve' analysis for lung volume in foetuses

2 lung_volume		Refresh	Categories	Help	
Name	**n**	**missing**	**min**	**max**	
1 id	173	0	1	52	
2 lung_volume	173	0	5,6	110,83	
3 weeks	173	0	17,71428	34,85714	
4 weeks_centred	173	0	-8,525014	8,617843	
5 cons	173	0	1	1	

From Output 6.12 it can be seen that 173 observations were made, and although it seems that these 173 observations concerned 52 'subjects', it must be realised that for three 'subjects' no measurements at all were made. Furthermore, it can be seen that not only the 'weeks' variable is present in the dataset, but also the 'weeks_centred' variable. In this situation it is recommendable to use the centred value of the 'time' variable, because the value of zero has no meaning at all. When the centred value is used, the intercept of the regression line will have a proper interpretation, i.e. the estimated lung volume at the average gestation age. The modelling process for this example will not be described in detail, but the final result is presented in Output 6.13.

Output 6.13. Results of a second-order multilevel 'growth curve' analysis for lung volume, with a random intercept and a random slope for the linear component of the number of weeks (centred)

$$\text{lung\_volume}_{ij} \sim N(XB, \ \Omega)$$

$$\text{lung\_volume}_{ij} = \beta_{0ij}\text{cons} + \beta_{1j}\text{weeks\_centred}_{ij} + 0,202\,(0,030)\,\text{weeks\_centred2}_{ij}$$

$$\beta_{0ij} = 31,638\,(1,260) + u_{0j} + e_{0ij}$$

$$\beta_{1j} = 4,554\,(0,176) + u_{1j}$$

$$\begin{bmatrix} u_{0j} \\ u_{1j} \end{bmatrix} \sim N(0, \ \Omega_u) : \Omega_u = \begin{bmatrix} 28,773(10,487) & \\ 6,472(1,579) & 0,513(0,317) \end{bmatrix}$$

$$[e_{0ij}] \sim N(0, \ \Omega_e) \ : \ \Omega_e = [80,403\,(11,182)]$$

$$-2*\text{loglikelihood}(IGLS) = 1266,595\,(173 \text{ of } 173 \text{ cases in use})$$

From Output 6.13 it can be seen that a second-order polynomial is the best way to describe the development of the lung volume over time. In other words, the Wald statistics for both the linear and the quadratic component of the 'time' variable (i.e. weeks_centred) are significant (a third-order component was also added to the model, but that did not resulted in a significant improvement of the model). It can further be seen that the model contains a random intercept and a random slope for the linear development over

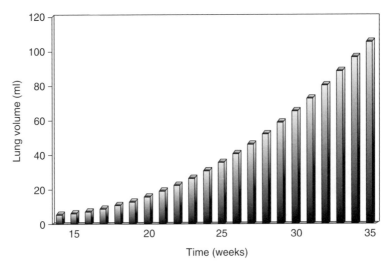

Figure 6.5. Graphic representation of the results of the 'growth curve' analysis for lung volume in foetuses.

time. A model with a random slope for the quadratic component of the time variable did not lead to a valid solution, so that component could not be added to the model. Although the regression coefficients can be interpreted directly, it is often more illustrative to present the results of such a growth curve analysis in a graph (see Figure 6.5).

For more detailed mathematical issues concerning growth curve modelling, reference is made, for instance, to Goldstein (1989a, b), Pan and Goldstein (1997), Huggins and Loesch (1998), and Stoel (2003).

6.5 Other techniques to analyse longitudinal data

Multilevel analysis is not the only technique that is available for the analysis of longitudinal data. Generalised estimating equations (GEE) is another technique that is frequently used (Zeger and Liang, 1986; Lipsitz et al., 1991; Zeger and Liang, 1992; Liang and Zeger, 1993; Twisk, 2003). The difference between multilevel analysis and GEE analysis, is that they each correct for the dependency of the observations in a different way. Multilevel analysis does so by allowing random regression coefficients, while GEE corrects by adding a so-called 'within-subject correlation structure' to the regression model. The advantage of multilevel analysis and GEE analysis is that they are both suitable for the longitudinal analysis of continuous as well as dichotomous and 'count' outcome variables. Another technique (which can only be performed in SAS software with the MIXED procedure), is comparable to GEE analysis, but different in that it does not add a 'within-subject correlation structure' to the regression model, but a 'within-subject covariance structure' (Littel et al., 1996, 2000). However, this technique is only suitable for the analysis of continuous outcome variables. It goes beyond the scope of this book to describe the various techniques in detail, but in order to assess the usefulness of multilevel analysis in longitudinal studies, it is important to describe briefly the similarities and differences in the results of longitudinal data analysis performed with the different techniques.

In general, when a continuous outcome variable is considered, multilevel analysis, GEE analysis, and the SAS method correcting for the 'within-subject covariance structure' give more or less the same results, although multilevel analysis is (probably) the most flexible of the three techniques. For dichotomous outcome variables, however, the situation is totally different. The regression coefficients of a logistic longitudinal multilevel analysis (i.e. a longitudinal multilevel analysis with a dichotomous outcome variable) are always higher than the regression coefficients obtained from GEE analysis. This means that the 'effects' estimated with multilevel analysis are more pronounced than those estimated with GEE analysis. However, the standard errors of the regression coefficients are also higher, so the significance levels are (theoretically) the same. One of the practical problems of logistic longitudinal multilevel analysis is that it seems to be very difficult to estimate the (random variances of the) regression coefficients, and therefore different estimation procedures lead to different results (see also Sections 4.2 and 9.3). The reason for the difference in results between multilevel analysis and GEE analysis is that multilevel analysis is a 'subject-specific' approach and GEE analysis is a 'population average' approach. For continuous outcome variables the results do not differ, but for dichotomous outcome variables multilevel analysis leads to higher regression coefficients. For a detailed discussion about the differences between multilevel analysis and GEE analysis, reference is made to Neuhaus et al., 1991; Hu et al., 1998; Omar et al., 1999; Crouchley and Davis, 2001; Twisk, 2003, 2004.

6.6 Comments

6.6.1 Extension of multilevel analysis for longitudinal data

The general idea of using multilevel analysis for the analysis of longitudinal data is to correct for the fact that the observations within individuals or patients are correlated. These correlated observations lead (in general) to correlated errors/residuals, which is the real problem in this kind of regression analysis. In most situations, allowing regression coefficients to differ between patients (i.e. allowing random regression coefficients) is enough to obtain uncorrelated errors/residuals. However, allowing random regression coefficients is sometimes not enough to correct for the correlated errors/residuals and an additional correction is needed. Therefore, in some software packages it is possible to perform an additional correction for either the 'within-subject correlation structure' or the 'within-subject covariance structure'. So, in fact, this additional correction combines more or less multilevel analysis with either GEE analysis (i.e. additional correction for the 'within-subject correlation structure') or the SAS MIXED procedure (i.e. additional correction for the 'within-subject covariance structure'). It is beyond the scope of this book to discuss this additional correction in detail. For additional information, reference is made to Pinheiro and Bates (2000), Rabe-Hesketh et al. (2001b, c), and Twisk (2003).

6.6.2 Clustering of longitudinal data on a higher level

In the examples discussed in this chapter, a two-level structure was considered. Repeated observations were clustered within patients. It is, of course, also possible that a three-level structure exists, e.g. repeated observations are clustered within patients and patients are clustered within medical doctors (see Figure 6.2). It should, however, be noted that when a three-level structure exists in a longitudinal study, GEE analysis and the SAS method correcting for the 'within-subject covariance structure' can no longer be used. Those two techniques are only suitable for a two-level structure. When a three-level structure exists in a longitudinal study, only multilevel analysis can be used.

6.6.3 Missing data in longitudinal studies

One of the biggest problems in longitudinal studies is missing data. There is an enormous amount of literature dealing with this problem (Little and

Rubin, 1987; Little, 1995; Schafer, 1997; Allison, 2001), most of which is related to the possible imputation of missing data to obtain a 'complete' dataset (Rubin, 1987, 1996; Shih and Quan, 1997; Schafer, 1999). However, when applying multilevel analysis to longitudinal data, there is no need to have a 'complete' dataset, and, furthermore, it has been shown that multilevel analysis is very flexible in handling missing data. It has even been shown that applying multilevel analysis to an incomplete dataset is even better than applying imputation methods (Twisk and de Vente, 2002; Twisk, 2003).

Multivariate multilevel analysis

7.1 Introduction

A special feature of multilevel analysis is that it can be used to perform multi-variate analysis. Multivariate analysis means that more than one outcome variable is analysed at one time. In the literature, multivariate analyses are often confused with multiple or multivariable regression analyses, in which the relationship between one outcome variable and more than one independent variable is analysed. That situation was discussed in Chapter 5. Multivariate analyses are not very common in medical science, but they are (for instance) widely used in psychology. Probably the most frequently applied multivariate technique is the multivariate analysis of variance (MANOVA), in which the average values of more than one continuous outcome variable are compared between groups. When a significant difference is found between groups, the next step is to examine which of the outcome variables differs between the groups, or, in other words, which of the outcome variables is related to the (group) determinant. When no significance difference is observed in multivariate analysis, this basically indicates that there is no significant relationship between the (group) determinant and the separate outcome variables as well. In this situation, the multivariate analysis can be seen as an efficient precursor of possible univariate analyses. When no multivariate relationship exists, univariate analysis does not necessarily have to be performed. When multivariate analyses is used in medical science, it is mostly used to analyse the relationship between one or more independent variables and a 'cluster' of outcome variables. In that respect, it is comparable with the so-called latent variable analysis, in which the 'cluster' of outcome variables are different aspects of a certain (not observable) latent variable. This kind of relationship is usually analysed with structural equation modelling (see, for instance, Jöreskog and Sörbom, 1993, 2001; Skrondal and Rabe-Hesketh,

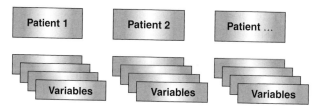

Figure 7.1. Two-level multivariate multilevel structure; variables are clustered within patients.

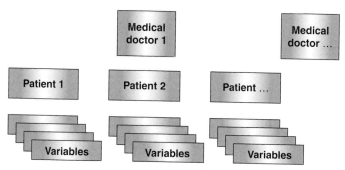

Figure 7.2. Three-level multivariate multilevel structure; variables are clustered within patients and patients are clustered within medical doctors.

2004). One of the problems with software packages for structural equation modelling, such as LISREL, EQS, or AMOS, is that they are very complicated, and far from user friendly. As has been mentioned before, multilevel analysis provides a very elegant alternative to perform a multivariate analysis (Rochon, 1996; Ten Have, 1996; Agresti, 1997; Catalano, 1997; Thum, 1997; Leyland et al., 2000; Gueorguieva and Agresti, 2001).

To perform a multivariate multilevel analysis actually means that below the level of the patient a 'variable' level must be created. So, comparable to the situation described in Chapter 6 for longitudinal data analysis, this will be a two-level structure with the different outcome variables as the lower level and the individual or patient as the higher level. Figure 7.1 illustrates this situation in which the outcome variables are 'clustered' within the patient. When the patients are further clustered (for instance) within medical doctors, this will result in a three-level structure (see Figure 7.2).

In the example in Chapter 2, the relationship between total cholesterol and age was analysed, and now this example will be extended with another outcome variable, i.e. systolic blood pressure. The research question of interest is whether there is a relationship between the 'cluster' of total cholesterol and

Table 7.1. Data structure needed to perform a multivariate multilevel analysis in MLwiN

Patient	Cholesterol	Systolic blood pressure	Medical doctor	Age
1	7.13	128	1	54
2	7.70	129	1	55
3	7.30	130	1	56
.				
.				
.				
n	4.10	127	12	46

systolic blood pressure, on the one hand, and age on the other. In fact, there are two ways in which this relationship can be analysed. The first way is incorporated in the MLwiN software, while the second one is a more general approach, and can be used in every software package that is suitable for performing multilevel analysis (see Section 7.3). Table 7.1 shows the data structure needed to perform a multivariate multilevel analysis in MLwiN.

7.2 Multivariate multilevel analysis: the MLwiN approach

Output 7.1 shows the descriptive information regarding the dataset used to illustrate a multivariate multilevel analysis in MLwiN.

Output 7.1. Descriptive information regarding the dataset used to illustrate multivariate multilevel modelling; the MLwiN approach

1 total cholester(		Refresh	Categories	? Help	
Name	n	missing	min	max	
1 total cholesterol	441	0	3,9	8,86	
2 systolic blood pressure	441	0	105	165	
3 medical doctor	441	0	1	12	
4 age	441	0	44	86	
5 id	441	0	1	441	
6 cons	441	0	1	1	

From Output 7.1 it can be seen that in addition to the variables that are already known (i.e. total cholesterol, medical doctor, age, id, and *cons*), systolic blood pressure is now also included in the dataset. Output 7.2 shows the results of a 'naive' multivariate analysis.

Output 7.2. Results of a 'naive' multivariate multilevel analysis of the relationship between total cholesterol and systolic blood pressure and age

$resp_{1jk} \sim N(XB, \Omega)$

$resp_{2jk} \sim N(XB, \Omega)$

$resp_{1jk} = \beta_{0j}cons.total\ cholesterol_{ijk} +$
$\qquad 0,051(0,004)age.total\ cholesterol_{ijk}$

$\beta_{0j} = 2,797(0,268) + u_{0jk}$

$resp_{2jk} = \beta_{1j}cons.systolic\ blood\ pressure_{ijk} +$
$\qquad 0,822(0,057)age.systolic\ blood\ pressure_{ijk}$

$\beta_{1j} = 75,302(3,580) + u_{1jk}$

$\begin{bmatrix} u_{0jk} \\ u_{1jk} \end{bmatrix} \sim N(0, \Omega_u) : \Omega_u = \begin{bmatrix} 0,696(0,047) & \\ 7,138(0,558) & 124,342(8,374) \end{bmatrix}$

$-2*loglikelihood(IGLS\ Deviance) = 4078,419(882\ of\ 882\ cases\ in\ use)$

From Output 7.2 it can be seen that there are two response variables ($resp_1$ and $resp_2$). Both are normally distributed, continuous outcome variables, and from the regression equations it is clear that the first response variable is total cholesterol and the second response variable is systolic blood pressure. After the regression equations, from which the relationship with age can be derived, a variance/covariance matrix is shown. It should be noted that this variance/covariance matrix does not give variances of the random regression coefficients (although the notation is u_{0jk} and u_{1jk}), but it only provides the variance/covariance error matrix. The error or residual variance is not a single value, but a matrix, because two outcome variables are analysed at the same time. Note that the error/residual in the output is represented by u (and not by e). Normally, u is used to indicate the variance of the random regression coefficients at the second level.

The last line of the output shows the -2 log likelihood. It can also be seen that there are *882 cases in use*. For each of the 441 subjects two observations are made; one for systolic blood pressure and one for total cholesterol. It is important to notice that two separate regression coefficients are estimated for the two outcome variables. The estimation of separate regression coefficients is 'recommended' in the multilevel user's guide (Rasbash et al., 2003). However, when separate regression coefficients are estimated it is not really clear what the advantage of the multivariate method is, compared to the separate univariate analyses, because they both give exactly the same results. Outputs 7.3 and 7.4 illustrate this.

Output 7.3. Results of a 'naive' linear multilevel analysis of the relationship between total cholesterol and age

---

total cholesterol$_{ij}$ ~ N(XB, Ω)
total cholesterol$_{ij}$ = β_{0i}cons + 0,051(0,004)age$_{ij}$
β_{0i} = 2,799(0,268) + e_{0ij}

[e_{0ij}] ~ N(0, Ω_e) : Ω_e = [0,696(0,047)]

-2*loglikelihood(IGLS Deviance) = 1091,752(441 of 441 cases in use)

Output 7.4. Results of a 'naive' linear multilevel analysis of the relationship between systolic blood pressure and age

---

systolic blood pressure$_{ij}$ ~ N(XB, Ω)
systolic blood pressure$_{ij}$ = β_{0i}cons + 0,821(0,057)age$_{ij}$
β_{0i} = 75,322(3,581) + e_{0ij}

[e_{0ij}] ~ N(0, Ω_e) : Ω_e = [124,349(8,374)]

-2*loglikelihood(IGLS Deviance) = 3378,486(441 of 441 cases in use)

The regression coefficients estimated from the 'naive' multivariate analysis could also be obtained from a 'standard' MANOVA (which can be performed in any software package). Output 7.5 shows the results of the

MANOVA with age as a covariate performed with SPSS. From Output 7.5 it can be seen that the results are exactly the same as the results shown in Output 7.2.

Output 7.5. Results of a MANOVA (performed in SPSS) to determine the relationship between total cholesterol and systolic blood pressure and age

Parameter Estimates

Dependent variable	Parameter	B	Std. error	95% Confidence Interval	
				Lower bound	Upper bound
Total cholesterol	Intercept	2,799	,269	2,271	3,327
	AGE	5,126E-02	,004	4,281E-02	5,971E-02
Systolic blood pressure	Intercept	75,322	3,590	68,267	82,377
	AGE	,821	,057	,708	,934

It is often argued that the advantage of using multivariate multilevel analysis is the possibility to estimate the association (or correlation) between outcome variables on different levels and in combination with independent variables. For instance, there is a big difference between the sum of the two -2 log likelihoods of the separate analysis for total cholesterol and systolic blood pressure (Outputs 7.3 and 7.4) and the -2 log likelihood of the multivariate analysis, in which total cholesterol and systolic blood pressure are analysed together. This difference reveals an association between the two outcome variables that can be interesting to investigate further. However, with multivariate multilevel analysis it is also possible to estimate one common regression coefficient for the outcome variables that are analysed together. Such a common regression coefficient indicates the relationship between the particular independent variable (i.e. age) and the 'cluster' of outcome variables. In my opinion, a multivariate multilevel analysis has especially interesting features when a common regression coefficient is calculated, although the interpretation of this regression coefficient is rather complicated. Output 7.6 shows the results of a 'naive'

Output 7.6. Results of a 'naive' multivariate multilevel analysis of the relationship between total cholesterol and systolic blood pressure and age, with one regression coefficient for age

---

```
resp₁ⱼₖ ~ N(XB, Ω)
```
$$\text{resp}_{1jk} \sim N(XB,\ \Omega)$$
$$\text{resp}_{2jk} \sim N(XB,\ \Omega)$$
$$\text{resp}_{1jk} = \beta_{0j}\text{cons.total cholesterol}_{ijk} + h_{jk}$$
$$\beta_{0j} = 5{,}56443\,(0{,}18548) + u_{0jk}$$
$$\text{resp}_{2jk} = \beta_{1j}\text{cons.systolic blood pressure}_{ijk} + h_{jk}$$
$$\beta_{1j} = 125{,}63760\,(0{,}66589) + u_{1jk}$$
$$h_{jk} = 0{,}00648\,(0{,}00292)\text{age.12}_{jk}$$

$$\begin{bmatrix} u_{0jk} \\ u_{1jk} \end{bmatrix} \sim N(0,\ \Omega_u)\ :\ \Omega_u = \begin{bmatrix} 0{,}86776(0{,}05839) & \\ 10{,}26362(0{,}77123) & 181{,}23890(12{,}20323) \end{bmatrix}$$

```
-2*loglikelihood(IGLS Deviance) = 4244,95700(882 of 882 cases in use)
```

---

multivariate multilevel analysis, in which one common regression coefficient is estimated for age.

The results shown in Output 7.6 are not very different from the results shown in Output 7.2. The only difference is the common regression coefficient in the latter analysis. The magnitude of this common regression coefficient of 0.00648 cannot be interpreted very easily because it is the relationship between age and the 'cluster' of outcome variables (i.e. systolic blood pressure and total cholesterol). However, what can be obtained from this output is that there is a significant relationship between age and this 'cluster'. As has been mentioned before, the significance of the regression coefficient can be obtained from the Wald statistic, i.e. the regression coefficient divided by its standard error squared. This value ($[0.00648/0.00292]^2 = 4.92$) follows a Chi-square distribution with one degree of freedom, which corresponds with a p-value of 0.03. The second step in the analysis is to evaluate whether or not the intercepts must be considered to be different for the medical doctors, i.e. whether or not random intercepts must be considered. Output 7.7 shows the results of that analysis.

From Output 7.7 it can be seen that the intercepts are considered to be random on the medical doctor level. In the output both intercepts are extended

Output 7.7. Results of a multivariate multilevel analysis of the relationship between total cholesterol and systolic blood pressure and age (one regression coefficient for age) with random intercepts

```
resp₁ⱼₖ ~ N(XB, Ω)
resp₂ⱼₖ ~ N(XB, Ω)
resp₁ⱼₖ = β₀ⱼₖcons.total cholesterolᵢⱼₖ + hⱼₖ
β₀ⱼₖ = 4,90033(0,23912) + v₀ₖ + u₀ⱼₖ
resp₂ⱼₖ = β₁ⱼₖcons.systolic blood pressureᵢⱼₖ + hⱼₖ
β₁ⱼₖ = 125,02730(2,26380) + v₁ₖ + u₁ⱼₖ
h₁ⱼₖ = 0,01729(0,00253)age.12ⱼₖ
```

$$\begin{bmatrix} v_{0k} \\ v_{1k} \end{bmatrix} \sim N(0, \ \Omega_v) \ : \ \Omega_v = \begin{bmatrix} 0,38131(0,16025) & \\ 4,49988(1,94760) & 57,86440(24,98637) \end{bmatrix}$$

$$\begin{bmatrix} u_{0jk} \\ u_{1jk} \end{bmatrix} \sim N(0, \ \Omega_u) \ : \ \Omega_u = \begin{bmatrix} 0,41675(0,02838) & \\ 5,02396(0,42102) & 122,60240(8,36920) \end{bmatrix}$$

```
-2*loglikelihood(IGLS Deviance) = 3995,96700(882 of 882 cases in use)
```

with a variance component (i.e. v_{ok} and v_{ik}). Note again that u_{0jk} and u_{1jk} reflect the error or residual variance, and not the variance of the random regression coefficient at the second level. The first variance/covariance matrix shown in the output is the matrix of the random intercepts. The importance of allowing random intercepts can be evaluated by performing the likelihood ratio test. Therefore, the difference between the −2 log likelihood of the model with the random intercepts and the −2 log likelihood of the model without the random intercepts must be calculated. This difference (4244.957 − 3995.967 = 248.99) is Chi-square distributed with three degrees of freedom, i.e. highly significant. Three degrees of freedom, firstly because of all the variances of the two intercepts are estimated, and secondly the covariance between the two intercepts is estimated. So, from the likelihood ratio test it can be concluded that it is important to allow the intercepts to differ between medical doctors. The relationship between age and the 'cluster' of systolic blood pressure and total cholesterol is highly significant. The regression coefficient is 0.01724, and the corresponding 95% CI ranges from 0.0071 to 0.0273. Again, there is no straightforward interpretation of the magnitude of this regression coefficient. The next step in the analysis is to

Output 7.8. Results of a multivariate multilevel analysis of the relationship between total cholesterol and systolic blood pressure and age (one regression coefficient for age) with both random intercepts and a random slope for age

---

$\text{resp}_{1jk} \sim N(XB, \ \Omega)$

$\text{resp}_{2jk} \sim N(XB, \ \Omega)$

$\text{resp}_{1jk} = \beta_{0jk}\text{cons.total cholesterol}_{ijk} + h_{jk}$

$\beta_{0jk} = 4,91041(0,41165) + v_{0k} + u_{0jk}$

$\text{resp}_{2jk} = \beta_{1jk}\text{cons.systolic blood pressure}_{ijk} + h_{jk}$

$\beta_{1jk} = 125,04310(2,39393) + v_{1k} + u_{1jk}$

$h_{jk} = \beta_{2k}\text{age.12}_{jk}$

$\beta_{2k} = 0,01724(0,00516) + v_{2k}$

$$\begin{bmatrix} v_{0k} \\ v_{1k} \\ v_{2k} \end{bmatrix} \sim N(0, \ \Omega_v) : \Omega_v = \begin{bmatrix} 1,70333(0,82549) & & \\ 8,75733(4,31775) & 65,10590(28,04546) & \\ -0,01804(0,00987) & -0,06629(0,04740) & 0,00024(0,00013) \end{bmatrix}$$

$$\begin{bmatrix} u_{0jk} \\ u_{1jk} \end{bmatrix} \sim N(0, \ \Omega_u) : \Omega_u = \begin{bmatrix} 0,41254(0,02828) & \\ 5,18920(0,42555) & 122,94080(8,39131) \end{bmatrix}$$

$-2*loglikelihood(IGLS\ Deviance) = 3974,18700(882\ of\ 882\ cases\ in\ use)$

---

allow the 'common' regression coefficient for age to differ between medical doctors. Output 7.8 shows the results of this analysis.

From Output 7.8 it can be seen that a random variance is added to the regression coefficient for age. The magnitude of this variance (i.e. v_{2k}) is given in the variance/covariance matrix of the random coefficients and is estimated as 0.00024. There are also two covariances between the two random intercepts and the random relationship with age. Both these covariances are negative, indicating that when the intercepts are high for a particular medical doctor, the relationship with age is weaker. The necessity of allowing a random regression coefficient for age can be evaluated by performing the likelihood ratio test. Therefore, the difference between the $-2\log$ likelihood of the model with a random slope and the model without a random slope must be calculated. This difference (i.e. $3995.967 - 3974.187 = 21.78$) follows a Chi-square distribution with three degrees of freedom, which has a p-value <0.001. The degrees of freedom is three because not only the random variance of the

Table 7.2. Data structure needed to perform an 'alternative', more general multivariate multilevel analysis

Patient	Outcome (z-score)	Medical doctor	Age	Variable
1	1.21	1	54	1
1	0.11	1	54	2
2	1.81	1	55	1
2	0.28	1	55	2
.				
.				
.				
n	−1.94	12	46	1
n	−0.06	12	46	2

relationship with age is estimated, but also the covariance of this random variance with the two random intercepts. Based on this p-value it can be concluded that a random slope for age must be considered. The difference between the analysis with and without a random slope for age is, furthermore, that the standard error for the regression coefficient for age is higher in the analysis with a random slope (which is not very surprising; see Chapter 3), while the magnitude of the regression coefficient remains roughly the same.

7.3 Multivariate multilevel analysis: the general approach

It has been mentioned before that there is also an 'alternative', more general way to perform a multivariate multilevel analysis. It must be realised that to perform this more general multivariate multilevel analysis, the outcome variables must be scaled in the same way. One of the possibilities is to calculate standardised values (i.e. z-scores) of the (two) continuous outcome variables under consideration. This means that from each total cholesterol observation, the average total cholesterol value has to be subtracted, and this value must be divided by the standard deviation of the total cholesterol values in the population under study. The same has to be done for the systolic blood pressure observations, with the average and standard deviation of the systolic blood pressure values. It should be noted that the data structure that is needed to perform the more general approach for multivariate multilevel analyses is different from the one described in Table 7.1 (see Table 7.2).

In the dataset illustrated in Table 7.1 there was one record for each patient, while in the dataset illustrated in Table 7.2 there are two records for each patient: one record for the total cholesterol values and one record for the systolic blood pressure values. Due to this, for the more general multivariate multilevel analysis there are 882 observations in the dataset to be analysed; i.e. two outcome variables for 441 patients. So, in fact, this kind of analysis is (really) comparable to longitudinal analysis, in which the same variable is measured over time. In a multivariate analysis, it is not the same variable that is measured within a patient, but different variables. Comparable to the situation in a longitudinal data analysis, the outcome variables measured on the same patients are correlated and that must be taken into account.

Output 7.9 shows descriptive information regarding the dataset used in this more general multivariate multilevel analysis.

Output 7.9. Descriptive information regarding the dataset used to illustrate multivariate multilevel modelling; the general approach

	Name	n	missing	min	max	
1	z_outcome	882	0	-2,148222	3,013231	
2	medical doctor	882	0	1	12	
3	age	882	0	44	86	
4	variable	882	0	1	2	
5	id	882	0	1	441	
6	cons	882	0	1	1	

From Output 7.9 it can be seen that there is only one outcome variable (called z_outcome) and that this outcome is measured 882 times; i.e. two outcome variables (total cholesterol and systolic blood pressure) for 441 subjects (see Table 7.2). As the outcome variables, total cholesterol and systolic blood pressure, are standardised (i.e. transformed into z-scores), the range of the outcome variable z_outcome is from -2.1 to 3.0. The fourth column of the dataset contains a variable named *variable*, which ranges between one and two and indicates which outcome variable is considered.

One stands for total cholesterol and two stands for systolic blood pressure. When a multivariate multilevel analysis is performed on this dataset, a three-level structure is considered. The lowest level is *variable* (subscript i), the second level is the patient (subscript j), and the highest level is the medical doctor (subscript k). Output 7.10 shows the results of a 'naive' analysis, in which the dependency of the observations within the medical doctor is ignored.

Output 7.10. Results of a 'naive' multivariate multilevel analysis of the relationship between total cholesterol and systolic blood pressure and age

```
z_outcome_ijk ~ N(XB, Ω)
z_outcome_ijk = β_0ij cons + 0,057(0,004)age_jk
β_0ij = -3,523(0,256) + u_0jk + e_0ijk

[u_0jk] ~ N(0, Ω_u) : Ω_u = [0,549(0,043)]
[e_0ijk] ~ N(0, Ω_e) : Ω_e = [0,170(0,011)]

-2*loglikelihood(IGLS Deviance) = 1826,110(882 of 882 cases in use)
```

From Output 7.10 it can be seen that the outcome variable is measured on three levels (subscripts i, j, and k). Furthermore, it can be seen that in this 'naive' analysis not only an error variance is estimated, but also a variance at patient level. This is because of the multivariate nature of the analysis. It should be noted that in this analysis not only a 'common' regression coefficient for age is calculated, but also a 'common' intercept. This differs from the method of multivariate multilevel analysis that was described in Section 7.2.

The second step in this analysis is to allow the intercept to differ between medical doctors, i.e. allowing a random intercept. Output 7.11 shows the results of this analysis.

From Output 7.11 it can be seen that the intercept is measured with three variance components: one variance component that indicates the variance at the medical doctor level (v_{0k}), one variance component that indicates the

Output 7.11. Results of a multivariate multilevel analysis of the relationship between total cholesterol and systolic blood pressure and age with a random intercept

---

```
z_outcome_ijk ~ N(XB, Ω)
z_outcome_ijk = β_0ijk cons + 0,057(0,003)age_jk
β_0ijk = -3,522(0,247) + v_0k + u_0jk + e_0ijk

[v_0k]  ~ N(0, Ω_v)  :  Ω_u = [0,349(0,146)]
[u_0jk] ~ N(0, Ω_u)  :  Ω_u = [0,204(0,021)]
[e_0ijk] ~ N(0, Ω_e) :  Ω_e = [0,170(0,011)]

-2*loglikelihood(IGLS Deviance) = 1525,382(882 of 882 cases in use)
```

---

variance at patient level (u_{0jk}), and the error or residual variance (e_{0ijk}). The magnitudes of these variance components are shown in the last part of the output. It can be seen that the variance of the intercept at patient level that was shown in Output 7.10 is now divided into two parts: one variance at patient level (i.e. 0.204) and one variance at the medical doctor level (i.e. 0.349).

When the $-2\log$ likelihood of this model is compared to the $-2\log$ likelihood of the model without the random intercept at the medical doctor level, it is obvious that it is necessary to allow the intercept to be random among the medical doctors (i.e. the likelihood ratio test is highly significant). In the next step, the model is extended with a random slope, i.e. the relationship between age and the 'cluster' of total cholesterol and systolic blood pressure is allowed to differ for different patients. Output 7.12 shows the results of this analysis.

From Output 7.12 it can be seen that the variance of the random slope at patient level is estimated as zero, and the same applies to the covariance between the random intercept and random slope. So, from Output 7.12 it can be concluded that a random slope at patient level must not be allowed (see Section 2.6.1). The last possible step in this analysis is to allow a random slope for the relationship between the 'cluster' of total cholesterol and systolic blood pressure and age on the medical doctor level. Output 7.13 shows the result of this analysis.

Output 7.12. Results of a multivariate multilevel analysis of the relationship between total cholesterol and systolic blood pressure and age with a random intercept at patient level and the medical doctor level and a random slope for age at patient level

$z\_outcome_{ijk} \sim N(XB, \Omega)$

$z\_outcome_{ijk} = \beta_{0ijk}cons + \beta_{1j}age_{jk}$

$\beta_{0ijk} = -3,522(0,223) + v_{0k} + u_{0jk} + e_{0ijk}$

$\beta_{1j} = 0,057(0,002) + u_{1jk}$

$[v_{0k}] \sim N(0, \Omega_v) : \Omega_v = [0,352(0,146)]$

$\begin{bmatrix} u_{0jk} \\ u_{1jk} \end{bmatrix} \sim N(0, \Omega_u) : \Omega_u = \begin{bmatrix} 0,000(0,000) & \\ 0,000(0,000) & 0,000(0,000) \end{bmatrix}$

$[e_{0ijk}] \sim N(0, \Omega_e) : \Omega_e = [0,371(0,018)]$

$-2*loglikelihood(IGLS\ Deviance) = 1679,533(882\ of\ 882\ cases\ in\ use)$

Output 7.13. Results of a multivariate multilevel analysis of the relationship between total cholesterol and systolic blood pressure and age with a random intercept at patient level and on the medical doctor level and a random slope for age on the medical doctor level

$z\_outcome_{ijk} \sim N(XB, \Omega)$

$z\_outcome_{ijk} \sim \beta_{0ijk}cons + \beta_{1k}age_{jk}$

$\beta_{0ijk} = -3,52233(0,31387) + v_{0k} + u_{0jk} + e_{0ijk}$

$\beta_{1k} = 0,05708(0,00490) + v_{1k}$

$\begin{bmatrix} v_{0k} \\ v_{1k} \end{bmatrix} \sim N(0, \Omega_v) : \Omega_v = \begin{bmatrix} 0,76326(0,47447) & \\ -0,00893(0,00683) & 0,00018(0,00012) \end{bmatrix}$

$[u_{0jk}] \sim N(0, \Omega_u) : \Omega_u = [0,19105(0,01995)]$

$[e_{0ijk}] \sim N(0, \Omega_e) : \Omega_e = [0,17004(0,01145)]$

$-2*loglikelihood(IGLS\ Deviance) = 1517,63900(882\ of\ 882\ cases\ in\ use)$

From Output 7.13 it can be seen that a random slope on the medical doctor level is added to the model. The regression coefficient for age is extended with a random variance at the medical doctor level (i.e. v_{1k}). The magnitude of this random variance is given in the first variance/covariance matrix shown in the output (i.e. 0.00018). The necessity of this random variance can be evaluated with the likelihood ratio test, in which the $-2\log$ likelihood of the model shown in Output 7.11 is compared to the $-2\log$ likelihood of the model shown in Output 7.13. This difference between the two $-2\log$ likelihoods is 7.743 (1525.382 $-$ 1517.639), which corresponds with a (two-sided) p-value of 0.02, when evaluated on a Chi-square distribution with two degrees of freedom. For the discussion of whether a one-sided or two-sided p-value must be used, see Section 2.2. The degrees of freedom is two because not only a random slope on the medical doctor level is estimated, but also the covariance between the random intercept and the random slope.

So, in conclusion, the last model is the best way to estimate the relationship between age and the 'cluster' of total cholesterol and systolic blood pressure. The regression coefficient for age in this model is 0.057, with a 95% CI ranging from 0.047 to 0.067, and a corresponding p-value <0.001. The magnitude of the regression coefficient can be interpreted in such a way that a difference of 1 year in age is associated with a difference of 0.057 standard deviation units in the 'cluster' of total cholesterol and systolic blood pressure. However, this interpretation is not really straightforward.

7.4 Comments

In this chapter, two ways in which to perform a multivariate multilevel analysis are discussed. In the example, a three-level structure was presented, but the 'standard' multivariate analysis deals with a two-level structure, i.e. the outcome variables are clustered within the individual or patient.

Although the two methods look different, both lead to comparable results. To illustrate this, the MLwiN approach is also used to analyse the relationship between age and the 'cluster' of standardised outcome variables. Output 7.14 shows directly the results of the 'final' analysis, in which both the intercepts and the relationship between the 'cluster' of standardised outcome variables and age are considered to be random.

Output 7.14. Results of a multivariate multilevel analysis of the relationship between total cholesterol and systolic blood pressure (both standardised) and age with random intercepts and a random slope for age (the MLwiN approach)

$\text{resp}_{1jk} \sim \text{N(XB, } \Omega\text{)}$
$\text{resp}_{2jk} \sim \text{N(XB, } \Omega\text{)}$
$\text{resp}_{1jk} = \beta_{0jk} \text{ cons.total cholesterol\_z}_{ijk} + h_{jk}$
$\beta_{0jk} = -3,53310(0,31157) + v_{0k} + u_{0jk}$
$\text{resp}_{2jk} = \beta_{1jk}\text{cons.systolic blood pressure\_z}_{ijk} + h_{jk}$
$\beta_{1jk} = -3,53236(0,31129) + v_{1k} + u_{1jk}$
$h_{jk} = \beta_{2k}\text{age.12}_{jk}$
$\beta_{2k} = 0,05724(0,00488) + v_{2k}$

$$\begin{bmatrix} v_{0k} \\ v_{1k} \\ v_{2k} \end{bmatrix} \sim \text{N (0, } \Omega_v\text{)} \; : \; \Omega_v = \begin{bmatrix} 0,74496(0,46646) & & \\ 0,72134(0,46059) & 0,74292(0,46570) & \\ -0,00829(0,00665) & -0,00894(0,00677) & 0,00018(0,00011) \end{bmatrix}$$

$$\begin{bmatrix} u_{0jk} \\ u_{1jk} \end{bmatrix} \sim \text{N (0, } \Omega_u\text{)} \; : \; \Omega_u = \begin{bmatrix} 0,35090(0,02423) & \\ -0,20241(0,01977) & 0,34886(0,02409) \end{bmatrix}$$

$-2*\text{loglikelihood(IGLS Deviance)} = 1476,28100 \text{ (882 of 882 cases in use)}$

The difference between the results reported in Outputs 7.13 and 7.14 is that in the first analysis two intercepts are estimated, while in the latter only one 'common' intercept is estimated. However, because both the outcome variables are standardised, the intercepts are almost the same for the two outcome variables. Therefore, the results reported in Outputs 7.13 and 7.14 are almost the same.

In the example, a multivariate problem was discussed, in which two continuous outcome variables were analysed together. The same procedures can be used when two or more dichotomous outcome variables are analysed together. However, when a combination of continuous and dichotomous outcome variables is analysed, the general approach in which to perform a multivariate analysis that was described in Section 7.3 cannot be used. On the other hand, the MLwiN approach described in Section 7.2 can be used to analyse combinations of any types of outcome variables.

It should be realised that the use of multilevel analysis for multivariate problems is not very common, and the advantages from this type of analysis, compared for instance to structural equation modelling, is still under investigation.

Sample-size calculations in multilevel studies

8.1 Introduction

Before performing an observational or experimental study, it is 'necessary' to calculate the number of subjects that are needed to make sure that a predefined effect will be statistically significant. It is 'necessary' because sample-size calculations are a prerequisite for research grants, and 'must' be submitted to (medical) Ethical Committees. Furthermore, for experimental studies, sample-size calculations are part of the so-called CONSORT statement. This means that, without a sample-size calculation, a paper reporting on the results of an experimental study will not be published. The importance of sample-size calculations is a rather strange phenomenon. Firstly, sample-size calculations are based on many assumptions, which can easily be changed, and in which case the number of subjects needed, will be totally different. Secondly, sample-size calculations are (usually) based on statistical significance, which is strange, because in epidemiological and medical research the importance of significance levels is becoming more and more questionable. However, many people believe in the importance of sample-size calculations, and because 'standard' sample-size calculations are not appropriate in multilevel studies, specific sample-size calculations for multilevel studies will be discussed in this chapter.

There is a considerable amount of literature on sample-size calculations in multilevel studies (e.g. Snijders and Bosker, 1993; Lee and Durbin, 1994; Liu and Liang, 1997; Cohen, 1998; Plewis and Hurry, 1998; Hedeker et al., 1999; Moerbeek et al., 2000, 2003c; Jung et al., 2001). In general, to calculate the number of subjects or patients needed in a multilevel study, first a standard sample-size calculation must be performed and then a correction factor must be added to it. The problem, however, is that there are two potential correction factors available, and that each leads to a (totally) different sample size.

8.2 Standard sample-size calculations

Standard sample-size calculations are basically designed for experimental studies. The expected difference between the intervention and control group in a certain outcome variable after the intervention is used as the effect size. Equation (8.1) shows the standard sample-size calculation for a continuous outcome variable:

$$N_1 = \frac{(Z_{(1-\alpha/2)} + Z_{(1-\beta)})^2 \times \sigma^2 \times (r + 1)}{v^2 \times r} \qquad (8.1)$$

where N_1 = sample size for the intervention group; α = significance level; $Z_{(1-\alpha/2)} = (1 - \alpha/2)$ percentile point of the standard normal distribution; $(1 - \beta)$ = power; $Z_{(1-\beta)} = (1 - \beta)$ percentile point of the standard normal distribution; σ = standard deviation of the outcome variable; r = ratio of the number of subjects in the groups compared, i.e. N_0/N_1; N_0 = sample size for the control group; and v = difference in mean value of the outcome variable between the groups.

For dichotomous outcome variables a comparable equation can be used (Equation (8.2)):

$$N_1 = \frac{(Z_{(1-\alpha/2)} + Z_{(1-\beta)})^2 \times \bar{p}(1 - \bar{p}) \times (r + 1)}{(p_1 - p_0)^2 \times r} \qquad (8.2a)$$

$$\bar{p} = \frac{p_1 + (r \times p_0)}{1 + r} \qquad (8.2b)$$

where N_1 = sample size for the intervention group; α = significance level; $Z_{(1-\alpha/2)} = (1 - \alpha/2)$ percentile point of the standard normal distribution; $(1 - \beta)$ = power; $Z_{(1-\beta)} = (1 - \beta)$ percentile point of the standard normal distribution; $\bar{p}$ = 'weighted' average of p_0 and p_1; r = ratio of the number of subjects in the groups compared, i.e. N_0/N_1; N_0 = sample size for the control group; p_1 = proportion of 'cases' in the intervention group; and p_0 = proportion of 'cases' in the control group.

8.3 Sample-size calculations for multilevel studies

As has been mentioned before, there are two different correction factors that can be used to calculate the required sample size in multilevel studies. Equation (8.3) shows the first correction factor:

$$m \times n = N \times [1 + (n - 1)\rho]$$
(8.3)

where N = number of subjects according to the standard sample-size calculation; m = number of 'clusters' (e.g. number of medical doctors, number of schools, etc.); n = number of observations for each 'cluster'; and ρ = intraclass correlation coefficient (ICC).

This factor is known as the 'design effect' and is mostly used in practice. It is also possible to calculate the relative 'effectiveness' of a certain sample size, when that sample size is applied in a multilevel study (Equation (8.4)):

$$N_{effective} = \frac{N}{[1 + (n - 1)\rho]}$$
(8.4)

where $N_{effective}$ = 'effective' sample size by a given 'standard' sample size (based on m times n observations).

Equation (8.5) shows the second correction factor that can be used to calculate the required sample size for a multilevel study. Equation (8.6) shows the corresponding equation to calculate the 'effective' sample size.

$$m = \frac{N}{1 + (n - 1)(1 - \rho)}$$
(8.5)

$$N_{effective} = m \times [1 + (n - 1)(1 - \rho)]$$
(8.6)

8.4 Example

Suppose that with a standard sample-size calculation it is calculated that 100 patients are needed in a certain experimental study, and that for each medical doctor 10 patients are included. Furthermore, let us assume that the ICC for patients within medical doctors is 0.2. When we add those figures to

Equation (8.3), it can be calculated that 28 medical doctors are needed; so instead of 100 patients, in a multilevel situation with a relatively small ICC of 0.2, 280 patients are needed. However, if we add those figures to Equation (8.5), it can be calculated that 12.2 medical doctors are needed, which means a sample size of 122 patients instead of 100.

If we calculate the 'effective' sample size in this situation (i.e. 100 patients, 10 medical doctors, and an ICC of 0.2), the 'effective' sample size calculated with Equation (8.4) is 35.7. According to Equation (8.6), on the other hand, the 'effective' sample size is 82.

8.5 Which sample-size calculation should be used?

The two procedures that can be used to calculate the sample size for a multi-level study lead to totally different results, and the questions arise that are which one is better and which one should be used? The first method that can be used to calculate the required sample size in a multilevel study (Equations (8.3) and (8.4)) can be characterised as a 'conservative' procedure, while the second method (Equations (8.5) and (8.6)) can be characterised as a more 'liberal' procedure. The way in which the two calculation procedures differ from each other can be best illustrated by a small example. Suppose the ICC in a certain multilevel study is 0.20. For the 'conservative' procedure this means that the first patient in a certain 'cluster' provides 100% new information, the second patient in that 'cluster' provides 80% new information. The third patient in that 'cluster' also provides 80% new information; however, not of the original 100%, but of the remaining 80%, which implies that the third patient only provides 64% new information. In the same way, the fourth patient in that 'cluster' only provides 51% new information (i.e. 80% of 64%), and so on. This implies that when the number of subjects increases for a certain medical doctor, almost no new information is obtained. As in the 'conservative' procedure, also in the 'liberal' sample-size calculation procedure the first patient provides 100% new information and the second patient provides 80% new information. However, the difference between the two procedures is that in the 'liberal' procedure all other patients in the 'cluster' also provide 80% new information. So, the third patient provides 80% new information, the fourth patient provides 80% new information, and so on.

To answer the question concerning which of the two methods is better, we can go back to Chapter 3, in which we discussed what was gained by using multilevel analysis. The example used in that chapter showed that in a 'naive' analysis with 100 patients an intervention effect of 0.289 was found, with a corresponding standard error of 0.121 (see Output 3.2). When random coefficients were allowed for both the intercept and the regression coefficient for the intervention, the magnitude of the intervention effect remained the same (i.e. 0.289), but the standard error increased to 0.175 (see Output 3.4). The ICC in this example was approximately 0.43. When the two sample-size calculation procedures are applied to this problem, according to the 'conservative' procedure 272 patients in the intervention group are needed to obtain the same efficiency/power as the 'naive' analysis with 100 patients. With the 'liberal' procedure only 155 patients are needed. Looking at the two standard errors of the 'naive' analysis and the multilevel analysis, it can be seen that the standard error in the 'corrected' analysis is 1.45 times higher than the standard error in the 'naive' analysis. If this is related to the increase in sample size, it means that $(1.45)^2 = 2.1$ times more patients are needed to obtain the same efficiency/power. In other words, 210 patients are needed in the intervention group in the 'corrected' analysis to obtain the same efficiency/power as in the 'naive' analysis. When these 210 patients are compared to the sample sizes estimated by the two equations, it can be seen that the 'conservative' method leads to an over-estimation, while the 'liberal' method leads to an under-estimation.

In the above example the randomisation was performed at patient level, but when the randomisation is performed at the medical doctor level (i.e. a 'cluster' randomisation), the situation is totally different. Let us go back to the example in Chapter 3, in which a 'cluster' randomisation was used, the results of which were summarised in Table 3.1. Outputs 8.1 and 8.2 show the results

Output 8.1. Results of a 'naive' analysis performed in MLwiN on a balanced dataset regarding the relationship between the intervention and health, when the randomisation was performed at the medical doctor level

```
health outcome_ij ~ N(XB, Ω)
health outcome_ij = β_0i cons + 0,259(0,121)intervention_j
β_0i = 6,517(0,085) + e_0ij

[e_0ij] ~ N(0, Ω_e)  :  Ω_e = [0,731(0,073)]

-2*loglikelihood(IGLS) = 504,849(200 of 200 cases in use)
```

Output 8.2. Results of a multilevel analysis on a balanced
dataset regarding the relationship between the intervention
and health, with a random intercept, when the randomisation
was performed at the medical doctor level

```
health outcomeᵢⱼ ~ N(XB, Ω)
health outcomeᵢⱼ = β₀ᵢⱼcons + 0,259(0,213)interventionⱼ
β₀ᵢⱼ = 6,517(0,151) + u₀ⱼ + e₀ᵢⱼ

[u₀ⱼ] ~ N(0, Ωᵤ)  : Ωᵤ = [0,171(0,072)]

[e₀ᵢⱼ] ~ N(0, Ωₑ)  : Ωₑ = [0,560(0,059)]

-2*loglikelihood(IGLS) = 479,544(200 of 200 cases in use)
```

of these analyses in greater detail. Output 8.1 shows the results of a 'naive'
analysis to estimate the intervention effect in this situation, while Output 8.2
shows the results of the corresponding multilevel analysis. Note that, because
the randomisation was performed on the medical doctor level only a random intercept could be allowed in this multilevel analysis.

From Output 8.2 it can be calculated that the ICC is approximately 0.23.
When this ICC is added to the sample-size equations, with the 'conservative'
procedure 307 patients are needed in the intervention group, while with the
'liberal' procedure only 126 patients are needed. From both outputs it can
further be seen that the intervention effect is equal (i.e. 0.259), but compared to the 'naive' analysis, the standard error of the intervention effect
increased in the multilevel analysis from 0.121 to 0.213, which is 1.76 times
higher. If this increase in the standard error is related to the increase in sample size, it means that $(1.76)^2 = 3.1$ times more patients are needed to
obtain the same efficiency/power in the multilevel analysis as in the 'naive'
analysis. In other words, when the randomisation is performed on the medical doctor level, 310 patients are needed in the 'corrected' analysis to obtain
the same efficiency/power as in the 'naive' analysis. So, in this situation the
'conservative' procedure is almost perfect, while the 'liberal' procedure leads
to a huge under-estimation of the required sample size.

In practice, the 'conservative' sample-size calculation procedure is mostly
used. However, most researchers do not realise that this procedure leads to

an overestimation of the required sample size when the randomisation is performed on the patient level.

8.6 Comments

It should be noted that with the sample-size calculations the number of clusters (i.e. noted as m) can be estimated. In most studies, however, the number of clusters (e.g. the number of medical doctors) that can be included in a study is not very flexible, and the question that must be answered is: how many patients should be included for each medical doctor? When using the 'conservative' procedure, there is a problem, because the sampling of more patients within a medical doctor is of little use. At a certain point (depending on the magnitude of the ICC) a new patient provides very little information. With the 'liberal' equation, sampling more patients for each medical doctor seems to be a potential way of increasing the efficiency/power of a multilevel study.

In fact, when designing a multilevel study, the most appropriate combination of the number of medical doctors and the number of patients within medical doctors must be calculated. In general, the more the medical doctors that are included in a study, the better. When the number of medical doctors is high in relation to the number of patients within medical doctors, there is less influence of the correlation between the observations within one medical doctor. However, it has already been mentioned that, theoretically, the most appropriate combination can be calculated, but in most practical situations this will be very difficult to achieve.

Finally, it should be realised that all sample-size equations presented in this section can be used to calculate the number of patients needed for an experimental study or to calculate the 'power' of that particular study. Again, it should be noted that for the sample-size calculations certain assumptions are necessary, i.e. with regard to the expected difference between the groups, the standard deviation of the outcome variable of interest, and the ICC. Furthermore, sample-size calculations are closely related to statistical significance. Due to these issues, the importance of sample-size calculations is rather limited, and therefore I believe that sample-size calculations should be used with great caution.

Software for multilevel analysis

9.1 Introduction

In the foregoing chapters, all examples of multilevel analysis were analysed in MLwiN. Although this software package is specially developed for performing multilevel analysis, there are also other software packages that can be used for multilevel analysis. In this chapter the example dataset(s) will be reanalysed with other software packages, and any differences in the results will be compared and discussed. For continuous outcome variables the research question concerned the relationship between total cholesterol and age (see Sections 2.2, 2.5 and 2.6.1), for dichotomous outcome variables it was the relationship between hypercholesterolemia and age (see Section 4.2), and for 'count' outcome variables the relationship between 'the number of risk factors' and age (see Section 4.4). For multinomial logistic multilevel analysis the population was divided into three groups, i.e. a group with relatively 'low' cholesterol values, a group with relatively 'moderate' cholesterol values, and a group with relatively 'high' cholesterol values (see Section 4.3). For linear multilevel analysis (i.e. multilevel analysis with a continuous outcome variable) both a two-level structure (i.e. patients clustered within medical doctors) and a three-level structure (patients clustered within medical doctors and medical doctors are clustered within institutions) will be used in the comparison. Only a two-level structure will be used for logistic multilevel analysis (i.e. multilevel analysis with a dichotomous outcome variable), for Poisson multilevel analysis (i.e. multilevel analysis with a 'count' outcome variable), and for multinomial logistic multilevel analysis (i.e. multilevel analysis with a categorical outcome variable). This chapter is limited in such a way that only the most commonly used software packages (i.e. SPSS, STATA, SAS, and R) will be described and compared to each other. There are other packages that can be used to perform multilevel analysis, such as MIXOR (Hedeker and Gibbons, 1996a), MIXREG (Hedeker and Gibbons, 1996b), HML (Bryk et al., 1999; Raudenbush et al.,

2001), SYSTAT (Hedeker et al., 2000), or EGRET (Cytel Software Corporation, 2000), but these will not be discussed in detailed here. For more information, and a comparison of software packages that can be used to perform multilevel analysis, reference is made to Goldstein (2004) and the corresponding web site.

9.2 Linear multilevel analysis

9.2.1 SPSS

Starting with version 11, SPSS provides the possibility to perform a linear multilevel analysis (i.e. a multilevel analysis with a continuous outcome variable). It should, however, be noted that SPSS version 11 is rather unreliable with respect to linear multilevel analysis. It is therefore recommended that at least SPSS version 12 is used for these analyses (Wolfinger et al., 1994; Landau and Everitt, 2004, O'Connor, 2004). Although SPSS is totally window driven, it is possible to run SPSS procedures by syntax. Multilevel analysis in SPSS is available under *mixed models*, and a linear multilevel analysis on the example dataset, with a continuous outcome variable with only a random intercept, can be obtained by running the SPSS syntax that is shown in Syntax 9.1.

Syntax 9.1. Syntax needed to perform a linear multilevel analysis, with only a random intercept, with the MIXED procedure in SPSS

```
MIXED
 tc WITH age
 /CRITERIA = CIN(95) MXITER(100) MXSTEP(5) SCORING(1)
           SINGULAR(0.000000000001)
HCONVERGE(0, ABSOLUTE) LCONVERGE(0, ABSOLUTE)
 PCONVERGE(0.0001, ABSOLUTE)
 /FIXED = age | SSTYPE(3)
 /METHOD = ML
 /PRINT = SOLUTION
 /RANDOM INTERCEPT | SUBJECT(md) .
```

The three most important lines in the SPSS syntax are the definition of the regression model (*tc WITH age*), the fact that a maximum likelihood estimation procedure is performed (*METHOD = ML*), and that only a random intercept is assumed on the medical doctor level (*RANDOM INTERCEPT | SUBJECT(md)*). All other information provided in the syntax is important for a proper analysis in SPSS, but is not really important enough to be explained in this book. It should be noted that in SPSS, restricted maximum likelihood is the default estimation procedure. Since a maximum likelihood estimation procedure was applied in the earlier examples, this was also done in the SPSS example. See Section 2.8.3 for the discussion regarding maximum likelihood and restricted maximum likelihood.

Output 9.1 shows (a selected part of) the results of a multilevel analysis, with only a random intercept, performed with the MIXED procedure in SPSS.

Output 9.1. Output of a linear multilevel analysis, with only a random intercept, performed with the MIXED procedure in SPSS

Mixed Model Analysis
Information Criteria[a]

-2 Log Likelihood	809,379
Akaike's Information Criterion (AIC)	817,379
Hurvich and Tsai's Criterion (AICC)	817,471
Bozdogan's Criterion (CAIC)	837,735
Schwarz's Bayesian Criterion (BIC)	833,735

The information criteria are displayed in smaller-is-better forms.
[a] Dependent Variable: total cholesterol.

Fixed Effects
Estimates of Fixed Effects[a]

						95% Confidence Interval	
						Lower	Upper
Parameter	Estimate	Std. Error	df	t	Sig.	Bound	Bound
Intercept	2,9058120	,2591340	52,539	11,214	,000	2,3859486	3,4256754
age	,0495866	,0030590	430,382	16,210	,000	,0435742	,0555991

[a] Dependent Variable: total cholesterol.

Covariance Parameters
Estimates of Covariance Parameters[a]

Parameter		Estimate	Std. Error
Residual		,3314923	,0226341
Intercept [subject = md]	Variance	,3685782	,1541986

[a] Dependent Variable: total cholesterol.

The first part of Output 9.1 gives the $-2\log$ likelihood. It has been mentioned before that this value can be used for the likelihood ratio test in order to evaluate whether or not random regression coefficients must be considered. Furthermore, the output shows some additional fit measures. All the additional fit measures can be seen as 'adjusted' values of the $-2\log$ likelihood, i.e. adjusted for the number of parameters estimated by the specific analysis. Akaike's Information Criterion (AIC) (Akaike, 1974) and Schwarz's Bayesian Information Criterion (BIC) (Schwarz, 1978) are the most frequently used fit measures. However, the way in which these measures are calculated is beyond the scope of this book.

The second part of Output 9.1 shows the regression coefficients, the 95% confidence intervals (CI), and the corresponding p-values. It can be seen from Output 9.1 that the p-value belonging to the (fixed) regression coefficients is derived from a t-test (rather than from a Wald test). Note that the number of degrees of freedom for this t-test is rather strange. However, because it is not really of great importance, the way in which the number of degrees of freedom is calculated will not be discussed any further. The last part of Output 9.1 shows the variance of the random intercept (i.e. 0.3685782) and the 'error' variance (i.e. 0.3314923).

To perform a random coefficient analysis, with both a random intercept and a random slope, Syntax 9.2 can be used.

Syntax 9.2 only differs from Syntax 9.1 in the last line, in which it is indicated that there is not only a random intercept, but also a random regression

Syntax 9.2. Syntax needed to perform a linear multilevel analysis, with a random intercept and a random slope for age, with the MIXED procedure in SPSS

```
MIXED
 tc WITH age
 /CRITERIA = CIN(95) MXITER(100) MXSTEP(5) SCORING(1)
            SINGULAR(0.000000000001)
HCONVERGE(0, ABSOLUTE) LCONVERGE(0, ABSOLUTE)
 PCONVERGE(0.0001, ABSOLUTE)
 /FIXED = age | SSTYPE(3)
 /METHOD = ML
 /PRINT = SOLUTION
 /RANDOM INTERCEPT age | SUBJECT(md) COVTYPE(UN).
```

coefficient for age. *COVTYPE(UN)* indicates that, in addition to a random intercept and a random slope, the covariance between the random intercept and random slope will also be estimated (i.e. to perform exactly the same analysis as has been performed with MLwiN in Section 2.5). Output 9.2 shows the results of this analysis.

Output 9.2. Output of a linear multilevel analysis, with a random intercept and a random slope for age, performed with the MIXED procedure in SPSS

Mixed Model Analysis
Information Criteria[a]

-2 Log Likelihood	799,963
Akaike's Information Criterion (AIC)	811,963
Hurvich and Tsai's Criterion (AICC)	812,157
Bozdogan's Criterion (CAIC)	842,498
Schwarz's Bayesian Criterion (BIC)	836,498

The information criteria are displayed in smaller-is-better forms.
[a]Dependent Variable: total cholesterol.

Fixed Effects
Estimates of Fixed Effects[a]

						95% Confidence Interval	
						Lower	Upper
Parameter	Estimate	Std. Error	df	t	Sig.	Bound	Bound
Intercept	2,8799320	,4010578	12,948	7,181	,000	2,0131464	3,7467177
age	,0500569	,0057599	10,765	8,691	,000	,0373456	,0627682

[a]Dependent Variable: total cholesterol.

Covariance Parameters
Estimates of Covariance Parameters[a]

Parameter		Estimate	Std. Error
Residual		,3136641	,0217537
Intercept +	UN (1,1)	1,4444621	,8473657
age [subject = md]	UN (2,1)	-,0171817	,0116309
	UN (2,2)	,0002724	,0001736

[a]Dependent Variable: total cholesterol.

From Output 9.2 it can be seen that four variance parameters are estimated (i.e. the random intercept ($UN (1,1)$)), the random regression coefficient for age ($UN (2,2)$), the covariance between the random intercept and the random slope ($UN (2,1)$), and the 'error' variance (*Residual*).

When a three-level structure is considered (i.e. patients clustered within medical doctors and medical doctors clustered within institutions), the syntax changes slightly (Syntax 9.3).

Syntax 9.3. Syntax needed to perform a linear multilevel analysis, with a random intercept on the medical doctor level and a random intercept on the institution level, with the MIXED procedure in SPSS

```
MIXED
  tc WITH age
  /CRITERIA = CIN(95) MXITER(100) MXSTEP(5) SCORING(1)
             SINGULAR(0.000000000001)
  HCONVERGE(0,ABSOLUTE) LCONVERGE (0,ABSOLUTE)
  PCONVERGE(0.0001, ABSOLUTE)
  /FIXED = age | SSTYPE(3)
  /METHOD = ML
  /PRINT = SOLUTION
  /RANDOM INTERCEPT | SUBJECT(md)
  /RANDOM INTERCEPT | SUBJECT(ins).
```

In the last two lines of Syntax 9.3 it is indicated that for both the medical doctor level and the institution level, a random intercept will be considered. Output 9.3 shows the result of this analysis.

Output 9.3. Output of a linear multilevel analysis, with a random intercept at the medical doctor level and a random intercept at the institution level, performed with the MIXED procedure in SPSS

Mixed Model Analysis

Information Criteria[a]

-2 Log Likelihood	799,827
Akaike's Information Criterion (AIC)	809,827
Hurvich and Tsai's Criterion (AICC)	809,965
Bozdogan's Criterion (CAIC)	835,272
Schwarz's Bayesian Criterion (BIC)	830,272

The information criteria are displayed in smaller-is-better forms.
[a] Dependent Variable: total cholesterol.

Output 9.3. *Contd.*

Fixed Effects

Estimates of Fixed Effects[a]

						95% Confidence Interval	
Parameter	Estimate	Std. Error	df	t	Sig.	Lower Bound	Upper Bound
Intercept	2,9161660	,3082930	15,184	9,459	,000	2,2597489	3,5725831
age	,0494219	,0030501	433,943	16,204	,000	,0434272	,0554166

[a]Dependent Variable: total cholesterol.

Covariance Parameters

Estimates of Covariance Parameters[a]

Parameter	Estimate	Std. Error
Residual	,3314968	,0226347
Intercept [subject = md] Variance	,0315255	,0234595
Intercept [subject = ins] Variance	,3371688	,2067390

[a]Dependent Variable: total cholesterol.

From the random variances shown in the last part of Output 9.3 it can be seen that at both the medical doctor level and the institution level a random intercept is considered.

9.2.2 STATA

Within STATA, the procedure General Linear Latent and Mixed Models (gllamm) can be used to perform multilevel analysis (Rabe-Hesketh and Pickles, 1999; Rabe-Hesketh et al., 2000, 2001b, c; Skrondal and Rabe-Hesketh, 2003b, 2004; Rabe-Hesketh and Everitt, 2004; Rabe-Hesketh et al., 2004). The procedure is very flexible (i.e. many different analyses can be performed), but it is also very time-consuming, and users need to be quite experienced. Furthermore, it is not available in the standard software package; it must be linked to the STATA software through a download from the Internet. The syntax needed to perform a linear multilevel analysis on the example dataset with only a random intercept is shown in Syntax 9.4.

Syntax 9.4. Syntax needed to perform a linear multilevel analysis, with only a random intercept, with the gllamm procedure in STATA

```
gllamm total_cholesterol age, i(medical_doctor) nip(12) adapt
```

The syntax to perform a multilevel analysis with the gllamm procedure is quite simple. First the procedure is called (*gllamm*), and secondly, the outcome variable (*total_cholesterol*) and the dependent variables are defined. In this example there is only one dependent variable: *age*. After the comma, the higher-level variable must be defined (i.e. *medical_doctor*). The last two parts of the syntax contain information regarding the estimation procedure used by gllamm. The command *nip* stands for the number of integration points and *adapt* stands for adaptive quadrature. There is no real rule for the number of integration points to be used in the analysis, but it is recommended that adaptive quadrature is always used (Rabe-Hesketh et al., 2002, 2004; Skrondal and Rabe-Hesketh, 2003b, 2004). It should be noted, however, that the result of the analysis highly depends on the number of integration points used, and on whether or not adaptive quadrature is used (Liu and Pierce, 1994; Lesaffre and Spiessens, 2001; Twisk, 2003).

Output 9.4. Output of a linear multilevel analysis, with only a random intercept, performed with the gllamm procedure in STATA

```
number of level 1 units = 441
number of level 2 units = 12

Condition Number = 123.75645

gllamm model

log likelihood = -404.6894
------------------------------------------------------------------------
total_chol~l │    Coef.  Std. Err.     z  P>|z|  [95% Conf. Interval]
-------------+----------------------------------------------------------
         age │ .0495891 .0030593  16.21 0.000   .043593    .0555852
        _cons│ 2.905732 .2591829  11.21 0.000  2.397743    3.413721
------------------------------------------------------------------------

Variance at level 1
------------------------------------------------------------------------
  .3315378 (.02263874)
Variances and covariances of random effects
------------------------------------------------------------------------

***level 2 (medical_doctor)
    var(1): .36880556 (.15436145)
```

Output 9.4 shows the results of a linear multilevel analysis performed with the gllamm procedure in STATA.

In the first two lines of Output 9.4 it can be seen that there are 441 *level 1 units* (i.e. patients) and that there are 12 *level 2 units* (i.e. medical doctors). In the next line *the Condition Number* is shown. This number is defined as: '*the square root of the ratio of the largest to smallest eigenvalues of the Hessian matrix*', and the explanation of this is far beyond the scope of this book (Rabe-Hesketh et al., 2001b, c, 2004). In fact, for non-experienced users this number is non-informative. Much more informative is the log likelihood that can be used for the likelihood ratio test. Again, it should be noted that the absolute value of the log likelihood is not informative, but only in comparison to the log likelihood of other (comparable) models. The next part of Output 9.4 contains information about the regression coefficients, and shows the magnitude of the regression coefficient, the standard error, the z-value (defined as the regression coefficient divided by its standard error), the corresponding p-value, and the 95% CI around the regression coefficient are shown. Note that in the gllamm procedure, the z-value is used to obtain the p-value of a certain regression coefficient. The z-value is comparable to the Wald statistic, because the Chi-square distribution with one degree of freedom is exactly the same as the standard normal distribution (z) squared.

The last part of the output shows the *variance at level 1* (i.e. the 'error' variance) and the *variance at level 2* (i.e. the variance of the intercepts for the different medical doctors), with their corresponding standard errors.

When a random slope is also considered for the relationship between total cholesterol and age, Syntax 9.5 can be used.

The first two lines of Syntax 9.5 are needed to define the random coefficients. First a random intercept is defined (*eq int: con*, where *con* stands for a variable with only ones; equal to the variable *cons* which is used in the MLwiN software), and secondly the random slope for age is defined (*eq slope: age*). The actual

Syntax 9.5. Syntax needed to perform a linear multilevel analysis, with a random intercept and a random slope for age, with the gllamm procedure in STATA

```
eq int:con
eq slope: age
gllamm total_cholesterol age, i(medical_doctor) nrf(2)
eqs(int slope) nip(24) adapt
```

command to run the gllamm procedure is extended with *nrf(2)*, which indicates that the number of random coefficients is two. With *eqs(int slope)* the two random regression coefficients are defined. Furthermore, the number of integration points in this example is 24, which is due to the fact that with 12 integration points the model did not converge, and therefore no solution was obtained.

Output 9.5 shows the result of a linear multilevel analysis, with a random intercept and a random slope for age, performed with the gllamm procedure in STATA.

Output 9.5. Output of a linear multilevel analysis, with a random intercept and a random slope for age, performed with the gllamm procedure in STATA

```
number of level 1 units = 441
number of level 2 units = 12

Condition Number = 212.35431

gllamm model

log likelihood = -399.9826
```

total_chol~1	Coef.	Std. Err.	z	P>|z|	[95% Conf. Interval]
age	.0500538	.0057937	8.64	0.000	.0386985	.0614092
_cons	2.880157	.4042767	7.12	0.000	2.087789	3.672525

```
Variance at level 1
----------------------------------------------------------------------
 .31368441 (.02175443)

Variances and covariances of random effects
----------------------------------------------------------------------
 ***level 2 (medical_doctor)
      var(1):  1.4709009 (.8663636)
      cov(2,1): -.01746172 (.01184719) cor(2,1): -.86687859
      var(2):  .00027585 (.00017602)
```

Most of Output 9.5 looks similar to what has been discussed for Output 9.4. The difference is in the last part of the output, where the random variances are shown. In the part *Variances and covariances of the random effects*, not only the variance of the random intercept (i.e. *1.4709009*) is shown, but also the variance of the random slope for age (i.e. *0.00027585*) and the covariance between these two (i.e. *−0.01746172*). In addition to the covariance, the corresponding correlation between the random intercept and the random slope is also shown (i.e. *−0.86687859*).

Syntax 9.6 shows the syntax that should be used to perform a three-level linear multilevel analysis with a random intercept at the medical doctor level as well as at the institution level.

Syntax 9.6. Syntax needed to perform a linear multilevel analysis, with a random intercept on the medical doctor level and a random intercept on the institution level, with the gllamm procedure in STATA

```
gllamm total_cholesterol age, i(medical_doctor institution)
nip(12) adapt
```

The only difference between Syntax 9.4 and Syntax 9.6 is that the level identification is extended with a third level, institution: *i (medical_doctor institution)*. Output 9.6 shows the results of the linear multilevel analysis with a random intercept at both the medical doctor level and the institution level.

Output 9.6. Output of a linear multilevel analysis, with a random intercept at the medical doctor level and a random intercept at the institution level, performed with the gllamm procedure in STATA

```
number of level 1 units = 441
number of level 2 units = 12
number of level 3 units = 6

Condition Number = 127.70098

gllamm model

log likelihood = -399.91377
```

total_chol~l	Coef.	Std. Err.	z	P>|z|	[95% Conf. Interval]	
age	.0494123	.0030514	16.19	0.000	.0434316	.055393
_cons	2.916848	.308367	9.46	0.000	2.31246	3.521236

```
Variance at level 1
```
```
.33148089 (.02263268)
```
```
Variances and covariances of random effects
```
```
***level 2 (medical_doctor)
    var(1): .03191509 (.02383943)
***level 3 (institution)
    var(1): .33705164 (.20682552)
```

The first part of Output 9.6 shows the three levels. The *number of level 1 units* = *441* (the number of patients), the *number of level 2 units* = *12* (the number of medical doctors), and the *number of level 3 units* = *6* (the number of institutions). The middle part of the output is comparable with what has been discussed before, and in the *Variances and covariances of the random effects* both variances of the random intercepts are shown, i.e. the variance of the intercepts at the medical doctor level (i.e. *0.03191509*) and the variance of the intercepts at the institution level (i.e. *0.33705164*).

It should again be noted that the results of all gllamm analyses highly depend on the number of integration points used, and on whether or not adaptive quadrature is used (Liu and Pierce, 1994; Lesaffre and Spiessens, 2001; Rabe-Hesketh et al., 2002; Twisk, 2003).

9.2.3 SAS

Within SAS, linear multilevel analysis can be performed with the MIXED procedure (Littel et al., 1991, 1996; SAS Institute Inc., 1997). Syntax 9.7 can be used to perform a linear multilevel analysis with only a random intercept with the MIXED procedure in SAS.

Syntax 9.7. Syntax needed to perform a linear multilevel analysis, with only a random intercept, with the MIXED procedure in SAS

```
PROC MIXED data = cont method=ml;
class md;
model tc = age/s;
random int /subject=md type=un;
RUN;
```

The syntax starts with the definition of the procedure for data analysis (i.e. PROC MIXED), and then mentions the dataset that must be used. Furthermore, the estimation method is set at maximum likelihood (*method* = *ml*). As with SPSS, the restricted maximum likelihood estimation procedure is the default, but for this example the maximum likelihood solutions from the different software packages are compared to each other. The second line of the syntax indicates that the medical doctor variable is a categorical variable, and the third line describes the model with only age as a determinant of total cholesterol. The */s* behind the model declaration is needed to print the solution.

The fourth line of Syntax 9.7 indicates that a random intercept must be considered (*random int*), and that the medical doctor variable indicates the second level (*/subject = md*). With *type*, different structures of the variance/covariance matrix of the random regression coefficients can be chosen. Note that this is not really necessary in a situation when only a random intercept is assumed. The last line of the syntax is necessary to run the analysis. Output 9.7 shows the results of this analysis.

Output 9.7. Output of a linear multilevel analysis, with only a random intercept, performed with the MIXED procedure in SAS

```
                    The Mixed Procedure

              Covariance Parameter Estimates

          Cov Parm     Subject     Estimate

          UN(1,1)        MD          0.3686
          Residual                   0.3315

                    Fit Statistics

     Log Likelihood                        -404.7
     Akaike's Information Criterion         -406.7
     Schwarz's Bayesian Criterion          -407.2
     -2 Log Likelihood                      809.4

           Null Model Likelihood Ratio Test

          DF     Chi-Square     Pr > ChiSq
           1       282.37         <.0001

              Solution for Fixed Effects

                        Standard
   Effect     Estimate    Error     DF   t Value   Pr > |t|

   Intercept   2.9058     0.2591     11    11.21     <.0001
   AGE         0.04959    0.003059  428    16.21     <.0001
```

The first part of Output 9.7 contains information regarding the random variance of the intercepts at the medical doctor level (*UN (1,1)*) and the residual variance. The second part of the output shows the -2 log likelihood of the model, and also a few fit measures that were also shown in the SPSS output (see Output 9.1). Again, both fit measures (*AIC* and *BIC*) are indicators of the likelihood that are adjusted for the number of parameters estimated by the model (Akaike, 1974; Schwarz, 1978). The last part of the output shows the regression coefficient for age (i.e. *0.04959*) with the standard error, the *t*-value and the corresponding *p*-value. So, like SPSS, SAS also uses the *t*-test rather than the Wald test to evaluate the significance level of a particular variable. However, the number of degrees of freedom for the *t*-test differs in the two software packages. For the intercept, the number of degrees of freedom is 11 (i.e. the number of medical doctors minus 1), while for age the number of degrees of freedom is 428 (i.e. the number of patients minus the number of medical doctors minus 1). Since the number of degrees of freedom for the regression coefficient for age is relatively high, the *t*-test and the Wald test lead to a similar result. It should be noted that Output 9.7 only shows a small part of the output generated by the MIXED procedure. Most of the output, however, is not really interesting.

Syntax 9.8 shows the syntax that is needed to perform a multilevel analysis, with both a random intercept and a random slope for age, with the MIXED procedure in SAS.

The difference between Syntaxes 9.7 and 9.8 can be seen in the fourth line where it is indicated that both the intercept and the age variable must be considered random at the medical doctor level (*random int age/subject = md*). The definition of the covariance structure is relevant in this situation, because two random variances and a corresponding covariance are estimated (see the software manual for a detailed description of the enormous amount of possibilities; Littel et al., 1991, 1996; SAS Institute Inc., 1997). An unstructured covariance matrix is chosen to obtain the same output as has been provided by MLwiN in Chapter 2. Output 9.8 shows (part of) the results of a linear multilevel analysis, with both a random intercept and a random slope for age, performed with the MIXED procedure in SAS.

Syntax 9.8. Syntax needed to perform a linear multilevel analysis, with a random intercept and a random slope for age, with the procedure MIXED in SAS

```
PROC MIXED data = cont method=ml;
class md;
model tc = age/s;
random int age /subject=md type=un;
RUN;
```

Output 9.8. Output of a linear multilevel analysis, with a random intercept and a random slope for age performed, performed with the MIXED procedure in SAS

```
                         The Mixed Procedure

                   Covariance Parameter Estimates

                 Cov Parm     Subject     Estimate

                 UN(1,1)        MD           1.4445
                 UN(2,1)        MD          -0.01718
                 UN(2,2)        MD          0.000272
                 Residual                    0.3137

                          Fit Statistics

             Log Likelihood                     -400.0
             Akaike's Information Criterion      -404.0
             Schwarz's Bayesian Criterion       -405.0
             -2 Log Likelihood                    800.0

                     Solution for Fixed Effects

                          Standard
  Effect        Estimate      Error     DF    t Value    Pr > |t|

  Intercept      2.8799      0.4011     11      7.18      <.0001
  AGE            0.05006     0.005760   11      8.69      <.0001
```

The difference between Outputs 9.7 and 9.8 can be found in the first part. In Output 9.8, not only the variance of the random intercepts (*UN (1,1)*, i.e. *1.4445*) is shown, but also the variance of the random slope for age (*UN (2,2)*, i.e. *0.000272*), and the corresponding covariance (*UN (2,1)*, i.e. −*0.01718*).

It should be noted that the number of degrees of freedom for the *t*-test to obtain the *p*-value for age is reduced to 11 (i.e. the number of medical doctors minus 1) when a random coefficient for age is considered. A reduction in degrees of freedom was also seen in the linear multilevel analysis performed with SPSS (see Outputs 9.1 and 9.2).

Syntax 9.9 shows the syntax that is needed to perform a three-level linear multilevel analysis, with random intercepts at both the medical doctor level and the institution level, with the MIXED procedure in SAS.

From Syntax 9.9 it can be seen that within the MIXED procedure in SAS, two lines are needed to define the random coefficients. In the first line the

Syntax 9.9. Syntax needed to perform a linear multilevel analysis, with a random intercept at the medical doctor level and a random intercept at the institution level, with the MIXED procedure in SAS

```
PROC MIXED data = cont method=ml;
class md ins;
model tc = age/s;
random int /subject=md type=un;
random int /subject=ins type=un;
RUN;
```

random intercept at the medical doctor level is defined (*random int /subject = md*), while in the second line the random intercept at the institution level is defined (*random int /subject = ins*). Output 9.9 shows (part of) the results of this linear multilevel analysis.

Output 9.9. Output of a linear multilevel analysis, with a random intercept at the medical doctor level and a random intercept at the institution level, performed with the MIXED procedure in SAS

The Mixed Procedure

Covariance Parameter Estimates

Cov Parm	Subject	Estimate
UN (1,1)	MD	0.03153
UN (1,1)	INS	0.3372
Residual		0.3315

Fit Statistics

Log Likelihood	-399.9
Akaike's Information Criterion	-402.9
Schwarz's Bayesian Criterion	-399.9
-2 Log Likelihood	799.8

Solution for Fixed Effects

Effect	Estimate	Standard Error	DF	t Value	Pr > |t|
Intercept	2.9162	0.3083	0	9.46	.
AGE	0.04942	0.003050	428	16.20	<.0001

It is not surprising that the difference between the three SAS PROC MIXED outputs can be found in the first part, in which the random variances are shown. From Output 9.9 it can be seen that there is a random variance of the intercepts at the medical doctor level (*UN (1,1) MD*, i.e. *0.03153*) and a random variance of the intercepts at the institution level (*UN (1,1) INS*, i.e. *0.3372*).

Although we are not really interested in the magnitude of the intercept, note that in the output table with the regression coefficients surprisingly no *p*-value of the intercept is shown (due to the fact that the number of degrees of freedom for the intercept is set at zero). However, the magnitude and the standard error of the intercept are comparable to what has been shown in all other packages.

9.2.4 R

R is a software package that has become increasingly popular in recent years. This is partly due to the fact that the software is free of charge and can be downloaded from the Internet (R Development Core Team, 2004). It is highly comparable to the S-plus software, and it basically uses the same programming environment (Venables and Ripley, 2000, 2002; Dalgaard, 2002; Fox, 2002; Maindonald and Braun, 2003). The difference between S-plus and R is that in R only syntax can be used, while in S-plus windows commands can be used for most procedures.

Multilevel analysis in R is provided by the glmmPQL procedure. Glmm stands for 'generalised linear and mixed models' and PQL stands for 'penalised quasi-likelihood', which was already seen in the MLwiN software. It should be noted that before the glmmPQL procedure can be used the MASS 'library' must be loaded (this can be done by typing: *require(MASS)*).

Syntax 9.10 shows the syntax needed to perform a linear multilevel analysis, with only a random intercept, with the glmmPQL procedure in R.

Syntax 9.10. Syntax needed to perform a linear multilevel analysis, with only a random intercept, with the glmmPQL procedure in R

```
model1 <- glmmPQL(tc ~ age, random = ~ 1|md, family=gaussian,
                  data=cont)
```

R is an 'object-oriented' programme, which means that the analysis should be linked to an object. The object for the first analysis is named *model1*. From Syntax 9.10 it can be seen that *model1* is linked to a glmmPQL analysis with total cholesterol as outcome and age as the only independent variable (*tc ~ age*). In the next part of the syntax the random regression coefficients are defined. In this example only a random intercept at the medical doctor level is assumed (*random = ~1 | md*). The last part of the syntax gives the dataset to be used (*data = cont*) and indicates that a continuous outcome variable must be analysed (*family = gaussian*). Output 9.10 shows (part of) the results of the glmmPQL analysis with only a random intercept. It should be noted that the results of the analysis are not directly shown; they are linked to *model1* and can be displayed by typing: *summary(model1)*.

Output 9.10. Output of a linear multilevel analysis, with only a random intercept, performed with the glmmPQL procedure in R

```
Linear mixed-effects model fit by maximum likelihood
 Data: cont
        AIC       BIC      logLik
    817.3788  833.735   -404.6894

Random effects:
 Formula: ~1 | md
          (Intercept)     Residual
StdDev:   0.6071064     0.5757537

Variance function:
 Structure: fixed weights
 Formula: ~invwt
Fixed effects: tc - age
                    Value    Std.Error    DF    t-value    p-value
(Intercept)   2.9058120   0.25972358   428   11.18810          0
age                   0.0495866   0.00306598   428   16.17319          0

Standardized Within-Group Residuals:
        Min           Q1          Med           Q3          Max
 -2.7893195   -0.7020637   -0.1437076   0.6559666   3.0894845

Number of Observations: 441
Number of Groups: 12
```

The first part of Output 9.10 provides the log likelihood of the model and two additional fit indicators derived from the likelihood (*AIC* and *BIC*). Both have already been explained in earlier Sections (e.g. Section 9.2.1). The second part of the output gives the standard deviation of the random intercept (i.e. 0.6071064). Note that R gives the standard deviation of the random regression coefficients, while most of the other software packages give the variance. The next part of the output gives the regression coefficients, the standard errors, the t-values, and the corresponding p-values. Note that also in R the t-distribution is used to obtain the significance level of the regression coefficient, and that the number of degrees of freedom is different from the number of degrees of freedom used in SAS (for the intercept) and SPSS (for both the intercept and the regression coefficient for age). In R the number of degrees of freedom is 428 (i.e. the number of patients minus the number of medical doctors minus 1) for both the intercept and the regression coefficient for age. The last part of the output shows the *Standardized Within-Group Residuals*. These can be used to check whether the residuals are normally distributed (see Section 2.7). Furthermore, the *Number of Observations* (i.e. patients) and the *Number of Groups* (i.e. medical doctors) are shown.

When the syntax is slightly extended, a multilevel analysis, with a random intercept as well as a random slope for the relationship between total cholesterol and age, can be performed (Syntax 9.11).

Syntax 9.11. Syntax needed to perform a linear multilevel analysis, with a random intercept and a random slope for age, with the glmmPQL procedure in R

```
model2 <- glmmPQL(tc ~ age, random = ~ age|md, family=
                  gaussian, data=cont)
```

The difference between Syntaxes 9.10 and 9.11 can be found in the definition of the random regression coefficients. In Syntax 9.11 both a random intercept and a random slope for age is assumed (*random = ~age|md*). Output 9.11 shows (part of) the results of this analysis.

As with the difference between Syntaxes 9.10 and 9.11, the only difference between Outputs 9.10 and 9.11 is found in the part that shows the standard deviations of the random regression coefficients. First the standard deviation of the random intercept is shown (i.e. 1.21050759), and then the standard deviation of the random slope for age (i.e. 0.01664172) and the covariance between the random intercept and the random slope (i.e. −0.868). Note again

Output 9.11. Output of a linear multilevel analysis, with a random intercept and a random slope for age, performed with the glmmPQL procedure in R

```
Linear mixed-effects model fit by maximum likelihood
 Data: cont
       AIC        BIC     logLik
  811.9642   836.4984   -399.9821

Random effects:
 Formula: ~age | md
 Structure: General positive-definite, Log-Cholesky
            parameterization
               StdDev      Corr
(Intercept)   1.21050759   (Intr)
age           0.01664172   -0.868
Residual      0.55995052

Variance function:
 Structure: fixed weights
 Formula: ~invwt
Fixed effects: tc ~ age
                 Value    Std.Error    DF    t-value   p-value
(Intercept)   2.8799294   0.4041667   428   7.125598        0
age           0.0500572   0.0058066   428   8.620751        0

Standardized Within-Group Residuals:
      Min          Q1          Med           Q3          Max
 -2.8541969   -0.6699815   -0.1145925   0.6222694   3.0848023

Number of Observations: 441
Number of Groups: 12
```

the difference in number of degrees of freedom between R, SAS, and SPSS for the *t*-test to obtain the *p*-value for the regression coefficients.

Syntax 9.12 shows the syntax needed to perform a three-level linear multilevel analysis with the glmmPQL procedure in R.

Syntax 9.12. Syntax needed to perform a linear multilevel analysis, with a random intercept at the medical doctor level and a random intercept at the institution level, with the glmmPQL procedure in R

```
model3 <- glmmPQL(tc ~ age, random = ~ 1|ins/md, family=
gaussian, data=cont)
```

Again, Syntax 9.12 only differs from Syntax 9.10 with regard to the defin-
ition of the random regression coefficients (*random* = ~1|*ins/md*). Output
9.12 shows part of the results of the analysis, with a random intercept at the
medical doctor level and a random intercept at the institution level, performed with the glmmPQL procedure in R.

Output 9.12. Output of a linear multilevel analysis, with a random intercept at
the medical doctor level and a random intercept at the institution level,
performed with the glmmPQL procedure in R

```
Linear mixed-effects model fit by maximum likelihood
 Data: cont3
       AIC        BIC       logLik
   809.8272   830.2725   -399.9136

Random effects:
 Formula: ~1 | ins
         (Intercept)
 StdDev:   0.5806615

 Formula: ~1 | md %in% ins
         (Intercept)    Residual
 StdDev:   0.1775394   0.5757582

Variance function:
 Structure: fixed weights
 Formula: ~invwt
Fixed effects:  tc ~ age
                 Value    Std.Error   DF    t-value     p-value
 (Intercept)   2.9161672  0.30899350  428   9.437633      0
 age           0.0494219  0.00305701  428  16.166736      0

Standardized Within-Group Residuals:
      Min          Q1          Med          Q3          Max
 -2.7323478   -0.7368539   -0.1309076   0.6559599   3.1321642

Number of Observations: 441
Number of Groups:
          ins md %in% ins
     6          12
```

From Output 9.12 it can be seen that two standard deviations of random
intercepts are estimated. The first one is the standard deviation for the
random intercept on the institution level (~1|*ins*, i.e. *0.5806615*) and the

Table 9.1. Overview of the results of a linear multilevel analysis, with only a random intercept, obtained from different software packages

	Age	Random variance intercept
MLwiN	0.0496 (0.0031)	0.3686
SPSS	0.0496 (0.0031)	0.3686
STATA	0.0496 (0.0031)	0.3688
R	0.0496 (0.0031)	0.3686
SAS	0.0496 (0.0031)	0.3686

second one is the random intercept on the medical doctor level ($\sim 1|md$ %in% ins, i.e. *0.1775394*). Furthermore, the output is comparable with what has been seen before, apart from the last line, which indicates that there were 12 medical doctors clustered within 6 institutions (*6 ins* and *12 md %in% ins*).

9.2.5 Overview

Tables 9.1–9.3 contain overviews of the results of the linear multilevel analyses obtained with the different software packages. Table 9.1 summarises the results of the linear multilevel analyses with only a random intercept. Table 9.2 summarises the results of the linear multilevel analyses with a random intercept as well as a random slope for the relationship between age and total cholesterol, and Table 9.3 summarises the results of the linear multilevel analyses with a three-level structure, i.e. with a random intercept at the medical doctor level and a random intercept at the institution level. In general, there is hardly any difference in the results of the different software packages; only marginal differences were observed in the random variances. It should, however, be noted that the three analyses that were performed are relatively simple, in such a way that only one independent variable was considered. Secondly, for a better comparison between the different software packages, the maximum likelihood estimation procedure was used for all software packages, while in some of the software packages, the restricted maximum likelihood estimation procedure is the default. Finally, when the gllamm procedure in STATA is used with a different specification of the number of integration points and with no specification of the adaptive quadrature, the results are totally different to those reported in this chapter.

Table 9.2. Overview of the results of a linear multilevel analysis, with a random intercept and a random slope for age, obtained from different software packages

| | Age | Random variance | |
		Intercept	Age
MLwiN	0.0501 (0.0058)	1.4426	0.0003
SPSS	0.0501 (0.0058)	1.4445	0.0003
STATA	0.0501 (0.0058)	1.4709	0.0003
R	0.0501 (0.0058)	1.4653	0.0003
SAS	0.0501 (0.0058)	1.4445	0.0003

Table 9.3. Overview of the results of a linear multilevel analysis, with a random intercept on the medical doctor level as well as on the institution level, obtained from different software packages

| | Age | Random variance intercept | |
		Medical doctor	Institution
MLwiN	0.0494 (0.0031)	0.0315	0.3372
SPSS	0.0494 (0.0031)	0.0315	0.3372
STATA	0.0494 (0.0031)	0.0319	0.3371
R	0.0494 (0.0031)	0.0315	0.3372
SAS	0.0494 (0.0031)	0.0315	0.3372

9.3 Logistic multilevel analysis

9.3.1 Introduction

It has already been mentioned in Chapter 4, in which logistic multilevel analysis (i.e. multilevel analysis with a dichotomous outcome variable) was explained, that it is mathematically rather difficult to perform a logistic multilevel analysis. However, except for SPSS, all other software packages discussed here (i.e. STATA, SAS, and R) provide the possibility to perform a logistic multilevel analysis.

9.3.2 STATA

With the gllamm procedure in STATA, in addition to linear multilevel analysis, logistic multilevel analysis can also be performed. In the syntax needed
to perform such an analysis it should be defined that the outcome variable is
dichotomous (see Syntax 9.13). This is done by specifying the so-called link
function (*link(logit)*) and specifying the distribution of the outcome variable (*fam(binom)*). It should be noted that, again, an adaptive quadrature is
specified. From the literature it is known that this is the estimation procedure that leads to the most valid results (Lessaffre and Spiessens, 2001; Rabe-
Hesketh et al., 2002; Rabe-Hesketh and Everitt, 2004).

Syntax 9.13. Syntax needed to perform a logistic multilevel analysis, with a
random intercept, with the gllamm procedure in STATA

```
gllamm hypercholesterolemia age, i(medical_doctor) fam(binom)
link(logit) nip(12) adapt
```

Output 9.13 shows the results of a logistic multilevel analysis with only a
random intercept performed with the gllamm procedure in STATA.

Output 9.13. Output of a logistic multilevel analysis, with a random intercept, performed
with the gllamm procedure in STATA

```
number of level 1 units = 441
number of level 2 units = 12

Condition Number = 160.24817

gllamm model

log likelihood = -180.74799
```

hyperchole~a	Coef.	Std. Err.	z	P>|z|	[95% Conf. Interval]	
age	.168253	.0210736	7.98	0.000	.1269496	.2095564
_cons	-11.29718	1.532116	-7.37	0.000	-14.30007	-8.294289

```
Variances and covariances of random effects

***level 2 (medical_doctor)
   var(1): 5.4880001 (2.7810829)
```

Output 9.13 is comparable to Output 9.4, in which the output of a linear multilevel analysis with a random intercept was shown. First the *number of level 1 units* is shown (i.e. number of patients) and secondly the *number of level 2 units* (i.e. number of medical doctors). The *condition number* and the *log likelihood* are also shown. Note that with MLwiN, no log likelihood could be estimated for a logistic multilevel analysis. This was due to the fact that in MLwiN a quasi-likelihood estimation procedure was used instead of a maximum (or restricted maximum) likelihood estimation procedure. The advantage of the gllamm procedure is, therefore, that different models can be compared to each other by means of the likelihood ratio test, which was not possible with MLwiN.

The last part of Output 9.13 firstly shows the regression coefficient for age (i.e. *0.168253*), the standard error, the *z*-value, the corresponding *p*-value and the 95% CI around the regression coefficient. It then shows the variance (and standard error) of the random intercept (i.e. *5.488001 (2.7810829)*). Due to the logistic nature of the analysis, the odds ratio for age can be obtained by calculating EXP[regression coefficient]. It is also possible to obtain the odds ratio directly by adding *eform* to Syntax 9.13.

9.3.3 SAS

For a linear multilevel analysis in SAS, the MIXED procedure could be used (see Section 9.2.3). However, with this procedure it is not possible to perform a logistic multilevel analysis. For such an analysis the NLMIXED procedure must be used. Syntax 9.14 shows the syntax needed to perform a logistic multilevel analysis, with only a random intercept, with the NLMIXED procedure.

Syntax 9.14. Syntax needed to perform a logistic multilevel analysis, with a random intercept, with the NLMIXED procedure in SAS

```
PROC NLMIXED data = dich;
parms beta0=-6.8 beta1=0.10 s2b0=1;
c1 = beta0 + b0;
eta = c1 + beta1*age;
expeta = exp (eta);
p = expeta / (1+expeta);
model hypertc ~ binary(p);
random b0 ~ normal ([0], [s2b0]) subject=md;
run;
```

Unfortunately, the syntax needed to perform a logistic multilevel analysis in SAS is rather complicated. As in all SAS procedures, the first line specifies the procedure and the dataset to be used. In the second line, the parameters to be estimated and their starting values must be specified. In this example there are three parameters to be estimated, the intercept (*beta0*), the regression coefficient for age (*beta1*), and the variance of the intercepts for the different medical doctors (*s2b0*). It should be noted that the results of the analysis highly depend on the chosen starting values. One of the possibilities to obtain starting values for the analysis is to perform a 'naive' analysis (i.e. an analysis that ignores the dependency of the observations within the medical doctors) and to use the results of that analysis as starting values for the logistic multilevel analysis with a random intercept. Of course, the starting value of the variance of the intercepts for the medical doctors cannot be obtained from the 'naive' analysis.

The next five lines of Syntax 9.14 show a rather complicated specification of the logistic model, while in the last line of the syntax it is specified that a random intercept is assumed and that the random intercepts are normally distributed (*random b0 ~ normal ([0], [s2b0])*), and that the random intercept is assumed at the medical doctor level (*subject = md*).

Output 9.14 shows (part of) the output obtained from a logistic multilevel analysis performed with the NLMIXED procedure in SAS.

Output 9.14. Output of a logistic multilevel analysis, with a random intercept, performed with the NLMIXED procedure in SAS

The NLMIXED Procedure

Fit Statistics

Description	Value
-2 Log Likelihood	361.5
AIC (smaller is better)	367.5
BIC (smaller is better)	369.0
Log Likelihood	-180.8
AIC (larger is better)	-183.8
BIC (larger is better)	-184.5

Parameter Estimates

Parameter	Estimate	Standard Error	DF	t Value	Pr > |t|	Alpha	Lower	Upper	Gradient
beta0	-11.2938	1.5308	11	-7.38	<.0001	0.05	-14.6630	-7.9246	2.958E-6
beta1	0.1682	0.02107	11	7.98	<.0001	0.05	0.1218	0.2146	0.000161
s2b0	5.4538	2.7513	11	1.98	0.0730	0.05	-0.6017	11.5093	7.192E-8

Compared to the complicated syntax, Output 9.14 looks quite simple, and is comparable to Output 9.7, in which the output of a linear multilevel analysis with a random intercept was shown. The first part of the output contains the *Fit Statistics*. Note that the NLMIXED procedure also uses a maximum likelihood estimation procedure, so it also provides a $-2\log$ likelihood that can be used to compare different models. The section *Parameter Estimates* contains the most important results of the analysis. This part shows the magnitude of the parameters defined in the second line of the syntax; *beta0* is the intercept, *beta1* is the regression coefficient for age, and *s2b0* is the variance of the intercepts for the different medical doctors. In addition to the magnitude of the parameters, it also shows the standard errors, the *t*-value, and the number of degrees of freedom for the *t*-distribution to obtain the *p*-value, the *p*-value and the 95% CI around the particular parameter. Note that the number of degrees of freedom is 11 (i.e. the number of medical doctors minus 1) for all parameters, which is different from the linear multilevel analysis. Note further that also the variance of the intercepts for the different medical doctors is evaluated by a *t*-distribution, which is rather strange (see Section 4.2). Finally, it should be noted that with the NLMIXED procedure in SAS, comparable to the gllamm procedure in STATA, adaptive quadrature is used to estimate the parameters of the model (Lesaffre and Spiessens, 2001).

9.3.4 R

Comparable to the difference in the syntax for the gllamm procedure in STATA, also in R only a slight change of the syntax shown in Syntax 9.10 is needed to obtain a logistic multilevel analysis instead of a linear multilevel analysis. It is not surprising that instead of *family = gaussian*, *family = binomial* must be typed (see Syntax 9.15). Output 9.15 shows the results of this logistic multilevel analysis with only a random intercept, performed with the glmmPQL procedure in R.

Output 9.15 looks similar to Output 9.10, in which the results of a linear multilevel analysis with only a random intercept were shown. First the *AIC*, *BIC*, and the *log likelihood* are shown. Note again that R, in contrast to MLwiN, but comparable to STATA and SAS, uses a maximum likelihood estimation procedure, and therefore provides a log likelihood which can be used to

Syntax 9.15. Syntax needed to perform a logistic multilevel analysis, with a random intercept, with the glmmPQL procedure in R

```
model4 <- glmmPQL(hyperch ~ age, random = ~1|md, family=
binomial, data=dich)
```

Output 9.15. Output of a logistic multilevel analysis, with a random intercept, performed with the glmmPQL procedure in R

```
Linear mixed-effects model fit by maximum likelihood
 Data: dich
        AIC       BIC      logLik
   2382.836   2399.192   -1187.418

Random effects:
 Formula: ~1 | md
          (Intercept)   Residual
StdDev:     2.220707   0.9020777

Variance function:
 Structure: fixed weights
 Formula: ~invwt
Fixed effects:  hyperch ~ age
                  Value   Std.Error   DF    t-value   p-value
(Intercept)   -11.022995  1.3503664  428   -8.162966      0
age             0.164433  0.0183055  428    8.982718      0

Standardized Within-Group Residuals:
       Min          Q1         Med         Q3        Max
  -6.6433638  -0.4749280  -0.1595897  0.3569172  5.8870434

Number of Observations: 441
Number of Groups: 12
```

compare different models. The second part of Output 9.15 shows the standard deviation of the intercepts for the different medical doctors (i.e. *2.220707*), and the third part of the output shows the magnitude of the regression coefficients. Note that the number of degrees of freedom for the evaluation of the *p*-value of the regression coefficient is different to the number used in the NLMIXED procedure in SAS. Although it is a remarkable difference, of course it does not have much influence on the magnitude of the *p*-value. The last lines of Output 9.15 (i.e. the *Standardized Within-Group*

Table 9.4. Overview of the results of a logistic multilevel analysis (i.e. with a dichotomous outcome variable), with only a random intercept, obtained from different software packages

	Age	Random variance intercept
MLwiN	0.180 (0.023)	5.590
STATA	0.168 (0.021)	5.488
R	0.164 (0.018)	4.932
SAS	0.168 (0.021)	5.454

Residuals) can (again) be used to evaluate whether or not the residuals are normally distributed (see Section 2.7).

9.3.5 Overview

Table 9.4 contains an overview of the results of a logistic multilevel analysis obtained from different software packages. Both the regression coefficients (including the corresponding standard errors) and the random variances differ (slightly) between the four software packages. It should be borne in mind that MLwiN uses a different estimation procedure (i.e. quasi-likelihood) compared to STATA, SAS, and R (i.e. maximum likelihood). It should further be noted that in STATA the results highly depend on the number of integration points, and whether or not adaptive quadrature was used. In SAS, the results highly depend on the starting values of the parameters.

9.4 Poisson multilevel analysis

9.4.1 Introduction

Poisson multilevel analysis (i.e. multilevel analysis with a 'count' outcome variable) can be performed with the same software packages that can be used for logistic multilevel analysis (i.e. STATA, SAS, and R). In fact, in most of the packages the difference in syntax between a logistic multilevel analysis and a Poisson multilevel analysis is that a different distribution of the outcome variable has to be specified. The dataset used in Section 4.4 is also used here to compare the different software packages. In that example dataset the relationship between 'the number of risk factors' (ranging from 0 to 5) and age was investigated.

9.4.2 STATA

Within STATA, like all other multilevel analyses, a Poisson multilevel analysis can also be performed with the gllamm procedure. Syntax 9.16 shows the syntax needed to perform a Poisson multilevel analysis with only a random intercept. The difference between the syntaxes needed for a linear multilevel analysis and a logistic multilevel analysis is that a different link function (*link(log)*) and a different distribution of the outcome variable must be specified (*fam(poisson)*).

Syntax 9.16. Syntax needed to perform a Poisson multilevel analysis, with a random intercept, with the gllamm procedure in STATA

```
gllamm number_of_riskfactors age, i(medical_doctor) fam
(poisson) link(log) nip(12) adapt
```

Output 9.16 shows the results of a Poisson multilevel analysis, with only a random intercept, performed with the gllamm procedure in STATA.

Output 9.16. Output of a Poisson multilevel analysis, with a random intercept, performed with the gllamm procedure in STATA

```
number of level 1 units = 441
number of level 2 units = 12

Condition Number = 205.89276

gllamm model

log likelihood = -556.82818

-----------------------------------------------------------------
number_of_~s |     Coef. Std. Err.    z   P>|z|  [95% Conf. Interval]
-------------+---------------------------------------------------
         age | .0238985  .0052921  4.52 0.000   .0135262    .0342708
        _cons| -1.662973  .357471  -4.65 0.000  -2.363603  -.9623425
-----------------------------------------------------------------

Variances and covariances of random effects
-----------------------------------------------------------------
***level 2 (medical_doctor)
    var(1): .13201919 (.06694393)
```

Output 9.16 looks very familiar, because it is comparable to the earlier outputs of the gllamm procedure. First the *number of level 1 units* and *the number of level 2 units* are shown, and secondly the *Condition Number* and the *log likelihood* that can be used to compare different models. Note that also for the Poisson multilevel analysis the gllamm procedure uses a maximum likelihood estimation procedure instead of the quasi-likelihood estimation procedure that was used in MLwiN. The second and third parts of the output show the regression coefficients (including the standard error, the *z*-value, the corresponding *p*-value, and the 95% CI around the regression coefficient) and the variance of the intercepts of the different medical doctors.

9.4.3 SAS

Within SAS, the NLMIXED procedure can be used to perform a Poisson multilevel analysis. The difference in syntax needed to perform this analysis and the syntax needed to perform a logistic multilevel analysis is that instead of the logistic model (see Syntax 9.14) a Poisson model is defined (see Syntax 9.17). All the rest is exactly the same. So, also for a Poisson multilevel analysis, starting values must be provided for all parameters that have to be estimated. As with the logistic multilevel analysis, it is recommended that the results of a 'naive' Poisson regression analysis are used as starting values for the Poisson multilevel analysis.

Syntax 9.17. Syntax needed to perform a Poisson multilevel analysis, with a random intercept, with the NLMIXED procedure in SAS

```
PROC NLMIXED data = pois;
parms beta0=-1.6 beta1=0.02 s2b0=0.1;
c1 = beta0 + b0;
eta = c1 + beta1*age;
expeta = exp (eta);
model riskfact ~ poisson(expeta);
random b0 ~ normal ([0], [s2b0]) subject=md;
run;
```

Output 9.17 shows the results of a Poisson multilevel analysis performed with the NLMIXED procedure in SAS.

Output 9.17 is comparable to Output 9.14 which showed the results of a logistic multilevel analysis performed with the NLMIXED procedure in SAS.

Output 9.17. Output of a Poisson multilevel analysis, with a random intercept, performed with the NLMIXED procedure in SAS

```
                                  Fit Statistics
                    Description                    Value
                    -2 Log Likelihood             1113.7
                    AIC (smaller is better)       1119.7
                    BIC (smaller is better)       1121.1
                    Log Likelihood                -556.8
                    AIC (larger is better)        -559.8
                    BIC (larger is better)        -560.6

                              Parameter Estimates

                    Standard
Parameter  Estimate    Error   DF  t Value  Pr > |t|  Alpha     Lower     Upper   Gradient
beta0       -1.6621   0.3573   11   -4.65    0.0007    0.05    -2.4486   -0.8757  -0.00561
beta1       0.02390  0.005291  11    4.52    0.0009    0.05     0.01226   0.03555  -0.33436
s2b0        0.1312   0.06640   11    1.98    0.0738    0.05    -0.01497   0.2773   -0.00793
```

Again, the output starts with the *Fit Statistics* (i.e. $-2\,Log\,Likelihood$, *AIC* and *BIC*), so again a maximum likelihood estimation procedure is used instead of a quasi-likelihood estimation procedure. The second part of the output contains the *Parameter Estimates*, and shows the estimates of *beta0* (i.e. the intercept), *beta1* (i.e. the regression coefficient for age), and *s2b0* (i.e. the variance of the intercepts for the different medical doctors). Note again that the p-values of all three parameters are estimated with a t-distribution with 11 degrees of freedom (i.e. the number of medical doctors minus 1).

9.4.4 R

As for all other multilevel analyses, the glmmPQL procedure in R can also be used for a Poisson multilevel analysis. The only difference is that a different family for the outcome variable must be specified, i.e. *family = poisson* (see Syntax 9.18).

Syntax 9.18. Syntax needed to perform a Poisson multilevel analysis, with a random intercept, with the glmmPQL procedure in R

```
model5 <- glmmPQL(numrf ~ age, random = ~1|md, family=
poisson, data=pois)
```

Output 9.18 shows the results of a Poisson multilevel analysis performed with the glmmPQL procedure in R. It is not surprising that the output looks similar to all other glmmPQL outputs shown before. First the *log likelihood* (as well as *AIC* and *BIC*) is shown and then the variance of the intercepts of the different medical doctors (i.e. *0.3540521*). The third part of the output contains the most important part of the results, i.e. it shows the regression coefficients, the standard errors, the degrees of freedom, the *t*-value, and the corresponding *p*-value. As with the logistic multilevel analysis, the *p*-value for the regression coefficients is derived from a *t*-distribution with 428 (i.e. the number of patients minus the number of medical doctors minus 1) degrees of freedom.

Output 9.18. Output of a Poisson multilevel analysis, with a random intercept, performed with the glmmPQL procedure in R

```
Linear mixed-effects model fit by maximum likelihood
 Data: pois
       AIC        BIC       logLik
  1408.793   1425.149   -700.3966

Random effects:
 Formula: ~1 | md
           (Intercept)     Residual
StdDev:     0.3540521     1.062121

Variance function:
 Structure: fixed weights
 Formula: ~invwt
Fixed effects: numrf ~ age
                    Value    Std.Error   DF    t-value    p-value
(Intercept)     -1.6441237   0.3771830   428   -4.358954        0
age              0.0238704   0.0056283   428    4.241175        0

Standardized Within-Group Residuals:
       Min           Q1          Med           Q3          Max
 -1.2643081   -0.7973350   -0.2148177   0.4748583   4.0556307

Number of Observations: 441
Number of Groups: 12
```

9.4.5 Overview

Table 9.5 contains an overview of the results of a Poisson multilevel analysis with only a random intercept obtained from different software packages.

Table 9.5. Overview of the results of a Poisson multilevel analysis (i.e. with a 'count' outcome variable), with only a random intercept, obtained from different software packages

	Age	Random variance intercept
MLwiN	0.024 (0.005)	0.131
STATA	0.024 (0.005)	0.132
R	0.024 (0.006)	0.125
SAS	0.024 (0.005)	0.131

It can be seen that this kind of analysis is rather robust, in that the results obtained from different software packages are almost the same. This is different from what has been seen for the logistic multilevel analysis (see Table 9.4), and it is rather remarkable because the different software packages use different estimation procedures. Quasi-likelihood is used in MLwiN, while maximum likelihood is used in STATA, SAS, and R.

9.5 Multinomial logistic multilevel analysis

9.5.1 Introduction

Multinomial logistic multilevel analysis (i.e. multilevel analysis with a categorical outcome variable) is a fairly new feature in standard software packages. Section 4.3 described the possibilities for performing such an analysis in MLwiN. At present, the only other alternative for multinomial logistic multilevel analysis is the gllamm procedure in STATA (Skrondal and Rabe-Hesketh, 2003a). In the example dataset, the outcome variable consists of three groups, i.e. a group of patients with relatively 'low' cholesterol values, a group of patients with relatively 'moderate' cholesterol values, and a group of patients with relatively 'high' cholesterol values (see Section 4.3). The research question of interest is whether the categorical outcome variable *cholesterol_group* was related to age?

9.5.2 STATA

Syntax 9.19 shows the syntax needed to perform a multinomial logistic multilevel regression analysis, with only a random intercept, with the gllamm procedure in STATA. From Syntax 9.19 it can be seen that only a different link function has to be specified (i.e. *link(mlogit)*), but the family that is specified is again binomial (i.e. *fam(binom)*).

Syntax 9.19. Syntax needed to perform a multinomial logistic multilevel analysis, with a random intercept, with the gllamm procedure in STATA

```
gllamm cholesterol_group age, i(medical_doctor) fam(binom)
link(mlogit) nip(12) adapt
```

Output 9.19 shows the results of a multinomial logistic multilevel analysis performed with the gllamm procedure in STATA. The output looks different to the earlier outputs of the gllamm procedure, in that the part of the output that shows the regression coefficients is double. The first part shows the regression coefficient for age, comparing the 'low' cholesterol group with the 'moderate' cholesterol group (i.e. *0.1341026*), while the second part shows the regression coefficient for age, comparing the 'low' cholesterol

Output 9.19. Output of a multinomial logistic multilevel analysis, with a random intercept, with the gllamm procedure in STATA

```
number of level 1 units = 441
number of level 2 units = 12

Condition Number = 1417.7473

gllamm model

log likelihood = -383.10378
----------------------------------------------------------------------------
cholestero~p :      Coef.  Std. Err.     z  P>|z|   [95% Conf. Interval]
----------------------------------------------------------------------------
c1           :
        age  :   .1341026  .0208802   6.42  0.000    .0931782    .175027
       _cons : -7.520526  1.346159  -5.59  0.000  -10.15895  -4.882103
c2           :
        age  :   .1918213  .0217325   8.83  0.000    .1492263   .2344163
       _cons : -11.25066  1.416899  -7.94  0.000  -14.02773  -8.473591
----------------------------------------------------------------------------

Variances and covariances of random effects
----------------------------------------------------------------------------
***level 2 (medical_doctor)
    var(1): 3.5814884 (1.9793861)
```

group with the 'high' cholesterol group (i.e. *0.1918213*). As in the logistic multilevel analysis, both regression coefficients can be transformed into an odds ratio by calculating EXP[regression coefficient]. The last part of the output again contains the variance of the intercepts of the different medical doctors. It can be seen that only one variance is shown (i.e. *3.5814884*), while in this situation MLwiN gives two variances, reflecting the variance of both intercepts (see Section 4.3, Output 4.9). A log likelihood is also shown for the multinomial logistic multilevel analysis (i.e. a maximum likelihood estimation procedure is used). Again, this is different from MLwiN, in which a quasi-likelihood estimation procedure is used.

9.5.3 Overview

Table 9.6 contains an overview of the results of a multinomial logistic multilevel analysis, with only a random intercept, obtained from STATA and MLwiN. For comparison, the results of a 'naive' multinomial logistic regression analysis (i.e. ignoring the dependency of the observations within the medical doctors) are also shown.

When the results of the two multinomial logistic multilevel analyses are compared, and also compared to the results of the 'naive' analysis, it is clear that there is a remarkable difference in estimated group 'effects'. Furthermore,

Table 9.6. Overview of the results of a multinomial logistic multilevel analysis (i.e. with a categorical outcome variable), with only a random intercept, obtained from different software packages

	Age	Random variance intercept
MLwiN		
Group 1	0.103 (0.011)	0.262
Group 2	0.172 (0.012)	1.392
STATA		
Group 1	0.134 (0.021)	
Group 2	0.192 (0.022)	3.581
SPSS (naive)		
Group 1	0.104 (0.017)	
Group 2	0.162 (0.018)	No random variance

it is surprising that with MLwiN the standard errors of the regression coefficients for age are lower than those obtained from a 'naive' analysis, while with STATA the standard errors of the regression coefficients are higher than those obtained from a 'naive' analysis. Although the latter seems to be more realistic, the difference between the results of a relatively simple analysis indicates that (at this point in time) one has to be very careful in interpreting the results of multinomial logistic multilevel analysis.

References

Agresti, A. (1997). A model for repeated measurements of a multivariate binary response. *Journal of the American Statistical Association*, **92**, 315–21.

Agresti, A., Booth, J.G., Hobert, J.P. and Caffo, B. (2000). Random-effects modeling of categorical response data. *Sociological Methodology*, **30**, 27–80.

Akaike, H. (1974). A new look at the statistical model identification. *IEEE Transactions on Automatic Control*, **19**, 716–23.

Albert, P.A. and Follman, D.A. (2000). Modeling repeated count data subject to informative dropout. *Biometrics*, **56**, 667–77.

Allison, P.D. (2001). *Missing Data. Series*. Thousand Oaks, CA: Sage Publications, Inc.

Atkinson, A.C. (1986). Masking unmasked. *Biometrika*, **73**, 533–41.

Barnett, V. and Lewis, T. (1994). *Outliers In Statistical Data*. New York: John Wiley.

Barthelemy, K.D. (2001). Modelling hierarchically clustered longitudinal survival processes with applications to childhood mortality and maternal health. *Canadian Studies in Population (Special Issue on Longitudinal Methodology)*, **28**, 535–61.

Baxter-Jones, A.D.G., Mirwald, R.L., McKay, H.A. and Bailey, D.A. (2003). A longitudinal analysis of sex differences in bone mineral accrual in healthy 8 to 19 year old boys and girls. *Annals of Human Biology*, **30**, 160–75.

Beunen, G., Baxter-Jones, A.D.G., Mirwald, R.L., Thomis, M., Lefevre, J., Malina, R.M. and Bailey, D.A. (2002). Intra-individual allometric development of aerobic power in 8 to 16 year-old boys. *Medicine and Science in Sports and Exercise*, **34**, 503–10.

Boyle, M.H. and Willms, J.D. (2001). Multilevel modelling of hierarchical data in developmental studies. *Journal of Child Psychology and Psychiatry*, **42**, 141–62.

Bryk, A.S. and Raudenbush, S.W. (1992). *Hierarchical Linear Models*. Newbury Park: Sage.

Bryk, A.S., Raudenbush, S.W. and Congdon, R. (1999). *HLM5: Hierarchical Linear and Nonlinear Modeling [Computer Software]*. Chicago: Scientific Software.

Carlin, J.B., Wolfe, R., Hendricks Brown, C. and Gelman, A. (2001). A case study on the choice, interpretation and checking of multilevel models for longitudinal binary outcomes. *Biostatistics*, **2**, 397–416.

Catalano, P.J. (1997). Bivariate modelling of clustered continuous and ordered categorical outcomes. *Statistics in Medicine*, **16**, 883–900.

Christiansen, C.L. and Morris, C. (1997). Hierarchical Poisson regression modelling. *Journal of the American Statistical Association*, **92**, 618–32.

Cohen, M.P. (1998). Determining sample sizes for surveys with data analyzed by hierarchical linear models. *Journal of Official Statistics*, **14**, 263–75.

Crouchley, R. and Davies, R.B. (2001). A comparison of GEE and random coefficient models for distinguishing heterogeneity, nonstationarity and state dependence in a collection of short binary event series. *Statistical Modelling*, **1**, 271–85.

Cytel Software Corporation. (2000). *EGRET for Windows, User Manual*. Cambridge, USA.

Dalgaard, P. (2002). *Introductory Statistics with R*. New York: Springer.

Daniels, M.J. and Gatsonics, C. (1997). Hierarchical polytomous regression models with applications to health services research. *Statistics in Medicine*, **16**, 2311–25.

Diez Roux, A.V. (2002). A glossary for multilevel analysis. *Journal of Epidemiology and Community Health*, **56**, 588–94.

Engel, B. (1998). A simple illustration of the failure of PQL, IRREML and AHPL as approximate ML methods for mixed models for binary data. *Biometrical Journal*, **40**, 141–54.

Fielding, A. (1999). Hierarchical random effects models for ordered category responses. In *Statistical Modelling: Proceedings of the 14th International Workshop*, eds. H. Friedl, A. Berghold and G. Kauerman, pp. 508–12. Technical University Graz, Graz, Austria.

Fielding, A. (2001). Scaling for residual variance components of ordered category responses in generalised linear mixed multilevel models. In *New Trends in Statistical Modelling: Proceedings of 16th International Workshop on Statistical Modelling*, eds. B. Klein and L. Korsholm, pp. 191–200.

Fielding, A., Yang, M. and Goldstein, H. (2003). Multilevel ordinal models for examination grades. *Statistical Modelling*, **3**, 127–53.

Fox, J. (2002). *An R and S-PLUS Companion to Applied Regression*. New York: Sage Publications.

Gerards, F., Twisk, J. and Vugt van, M.G. (2004). Fetal lung volume measured by 3-dimensional ultrasound in pregnancies suspected for pulmonary hypoplasia. *Ultrasound in Obstetrics and Gynecology*, **24**, 233.

Gerards, F.A., Engels, M.A.J., Twisk, J.W.R. and Vugt van, J.M.G. (2005). Normal fetal lung volume measured with 3-dimensional ultrasonography (3D fetal lung volume). Submitted for publication.

Goldstein, H. (1987). *Multilevel Models in Educational and Social Research*. London, Griffin; New York: Oxford University Press.

Goldstein, H. and Cuttance, P. (1988). A note on national assessment and school comparisons. *Journal of Education Policy*, **3**, 197–202.

Goldstein, H. (1989a). Flexible models for the analysis of growth data with an application to height prediction. *Revue de Epidemiology et Sante Public*, **37**, 477–84.

Goldstein, H. (1989b). Models for multilevel response variables with an application to growth curves. *Multilevel Analysis of Educational Data*, ed. R.D. Bock, pp. 107–25. New York: Academic Press.

Goldstein, H. (1992). Statistical information and the measurement of education outcomes (editorial). *Journal of the Royal Statistical Society, A*, **155**, 313–15.

Goldstein, H. and Healy, M.J.R. (1995). The graphical presentation of a collection of means. *Journal of the Royal Statistical Society, A*, **158**, 175–7.

Goldstein, H. (1995). *Multilevel Statistical Models*. London: Edward Arnold.

Goldstein, H. and Spiegelhalter, D.J. (1996). League tables and their limitations: statistical issues in comparisons of institutional performance. *Journal of the Royal Statistical Society, A*, **159**, 385–443.

Goldstein, H. and Rasbash, J. (1996). Improved approximation for multilevel models with binary responses. *Journal of the Royal Statistical Society*, **159**, 505–13.

Goldstein, H., Rasbash, J., Plewis, I., Draper, D., Browne, W., Yang, M., Woodhouse, G. and Healy, M. (1998). *A User's Guide to MLwiN*. London: Institute of Education.

Goldstein, H. (2003). *Multilevel Statistical Models*, 3rd edition. London: Edward Arnold.

Goldstein, H. (2004). A review of multilevel software packages. *Multilevel Modelling Newsletter*, **16**, 18–19 (http://multilevel.ioe.ac.uk/softrev/index.html).

Greenland, S. (1997). Second stage least squares versus penalized quasi-likelihood for fitting hierarchical models in epidemiologic analysis. *Statistics in Medicine*, **16**, 515–26.

Greenland, S. (2000a). When should epidemiologic regressions use random coefficients? *Biometrics*, **56**, 915–21.

Greenland, S. (2000b). Principles of multilevel modelling. *International Journal of Epidemiology*, **29**, 158–67.

Grilli, L. and Rampichini, C. (2003). Alternative specifications of multivariate multilevel probit ordinal response models. *Journal of Educational and Behavioral Statistics*, **28**, 31–44.

Gueorguieva, R.V. and Agresti, A. (2001). A correlated probit model for joint modelling of clustered binary and continuous responses. *Journal of the American Statistical Association*, **96**, 1102–12.

Hedeker, D. and Gibbons, R.D. (1996a). MIXOR: a computer program for mixed effects ordinal regression analysis. *Computer Methods and Programs in Biomedicine*, **49**, 157–76.

Hedeker, D. and Gibbons, R.D. (1996b). MIXREG: a computer program for mixed-effects regression analysis with autocorrelated errors. *Computer Methods and Programs in Biomedicine*, **49**, 229–52.

Hedeker, D., Gibbons, R.D. and Waternaux, C. (1999). Sample size estimation for longitudinal designs with attrition: comparing time-related contrasts between groups. *Journal of Education and Behavioral Statistics*, **24**, 70–93.

Hedeker, D., Marcantonio, R. and Pechnyo, M. (2000). *Chapter 2: Mixed Regression*. SYSTAT 10, Statistics II.

Heo, M., Faith, M.S., Mott, J.W., Gorman, B.S., Redden, D.T. and Allison, D.B. (2003). Hierarchical linear models for the development of growth curves: an example with body mass index in overweight/obese adults. *Statistics in Medicine*, **22**, 1911–42.

Hernández-Lloreda, M.V., Colmenares, F. and Martínez-Arias, R. (2003). Application of hierarchical linear modelling to the study of trajectories of behavioural development. *Animal Behaviour*, **65**, 607–13.

Hogan, J.W. and Laird, N.M. (1997). Mixture models for the joint distribution of repeated measurements and event times. *Statistics in Medicine*, **16**, 239–58.

Hox, J.J. (1995). *Applied Multilevel Analysis*. Amsterdam: T-T Publikaties.

Hox, J.J. (2002). *Multilevel Analysis. Techniques and Applications*. Mahwah, NJ: Lawrence Erlbaum Associates.

Hu, F.B., Goldberg, J., Hedeker, D., Flay, B.R. and Pentz, M.A. (1998). Comparison of population-averaged and subject specific approaches for analyzing repeated measures binary outcomes. *American Journal of Epidemiology*, 147, 694–703.

Huggins, R.M. and Loesch, D.Z. (1998). On the analysis of mixed longitudinal growth data. *Biometrics*, 54, 583–95.

Hutchinson, D. and Healy, M. (2001). The effect of variance component estimates of ignoring a level in a multilevel model. *Multilevel Modelling Newsletter*, 13, 4–5.

Jöreskog, K.G. and Sörbom, D. (1993). *LISREL 8 User's Reference Guide*. Chicago, IL: Scientific Software International.

Jöreskog, K.G. and Sörbom, D. (2001). *LISREL 8.5*. Chicago, IL: Scientific Software International.

Jung, S.H., Kang, S.H. and Ahn, C. (2001). Sample size calculations for clustered binary data. *Statistics in Medicine*, 20, 1971–82.

Korff, von, M., Koepsell, T., Curry, S. and Diehr, P. (1992). Multilevel analysis in epidemiologic research on health behaviors and outcomes. *American Journal of Epidemiology*, 135, 1077–82.

Kreft, I. and Leeuw de, J. (1998). *Introducing Multilevel Modelling*. London: Sage Publications.

Langford, I.H. and Lewis, T. (1998). Outliers in multilevel models (with discussion). *Journal of the Royal Statistical Society, A*, 161, 121–60.

Landau, S. and Everitt, B.S. (2004). *A handbook of statistical analysis using SPSS*. Boca Raton: Chapman & Hall.

Larsen, K., Petersen, J.H., Budtz-Jorgensen, E. and Endahl, L. (2000). Interpreting parameters in the logistic regression model with random effects. *Biometrics*, 56, 909–14.

Larsen, K. and Merlo, J. (2005). Appropriate assessment of neighborhood effects on individual health: integrating random and fixed effects in multilevel logistic regression: *American Journal of Epidemiology*, 161, 81–88.

Lawrence, A.J. (1995). Deletion, influence and masking in regression. *Journal of the Royal Statistical Society, B*, 57, 181–89.

Lee, E.W. and Durbin, N. (1994). Estimation and sample size considerations for clustered binary responses. *Statistics in Medicine*, 13, 1241–52.

Lesaffre, E. and Spiessens, B. (2001). On the effect of the number of quadrature points in a logistic random-effects model: an example. *Applied Statistics*, 50, 325–35.

Leyland, A.H., Langford, I.H., Rasbash, J. and Goldstein, H. (2000). Multivariate spatial models for event data. *Statistics in Medicine*, 19, 2469–78.

Leyland, A.H. and Groenewegen, P.P. (2003). Multilevel modelling and public health policy. *Scandinavian Journal of Public Health*, 31, 267–74.

Liang, K.-Y. and Zeger, S.L. (1993). Regression analysis for correlated data. *Annual Review of Public Health*, 14, 43–68.

Lin, X. (1997). Variance component testing in generalised linear models with random effects. *Biometrika*, 84, 309–25.

Lipsitz, S.R., Laird, N.M. and Harrington, D.P. (1991). Generalized estimating equations for correlated binary data: using the odds ratio as a measure of association. *Biometrika*, 78, 153–60.

Littel, R.C., Freund, R.J. and Spector, P.C. (1991). *SAS System for Linear Models*, 3rd edition. Cary NC: SAS Institute Inc.

Littel, R.C., Milliken, G.A., Stroup, W.W. and Wolfinger, R.D. (1996). *SAS System for Mixed Models*. Cary, NC: SAS Institute Inc.

Littel, R.C., Pendergast, J. and Natarajan, R. (2000). Modelling covariance structures in the analysis of repeated measures data. *Statistics in Medicine*, **19**, 1793–819.

Little, R.J.A. and Rubin, D.B. (1987). *Statistical Analysis with Missing Data*. New York: John Wiley.

Little, R.J.A. (1995). Modelling the drop-out mechanism repeated measures studies. *Journal of the American Statistical Association*, **90**, 1112–21.

Little, T.D., Schabel, K.U. and Baumert, J. (Eds). (2000). *Modeling Longitudinal and Multilevel Data: Practical Issues, Applies Approaches, and Specific Examples*. Mahwah: Lawrence Erlbaum.

Liu, Q. and Pierce, D.A. (1994). A note on Gauss-Hermite quadrature. *Biometrika*, **81**, 624–9.

Liu, G. and Liang, K.-Y. (1997). Sample size calculations for studies with correlated observations. *Biometrics*, **53**, 937–47.

Livert, D., Rindskopf, D., Saxe, L. and Stirratt, M. (2001). Using multilevel modelling in the evaluation of community-based treatment programs. *Multivariate Behavioral Research*, **36**, 155–83.

Maindonald, J. and Braun, J. (2003). *Data Analysis and Graphics Using R: An Example-based Approach*. Cambridge: Cambridge University Press.

McCullagh, P. and Searle, S.R. (2001). *Generalized, Linear and Mixed Models*. New York: Wiley.

Mealli, F. and Rampichini, C. (1999). Estimating binary multilevel models through indirect inference. *Computational Statistics and Data Analysis*, **29**, 313–24.

Merlo, J., Östergren, P.-O., Broms, K., Bjorck-Linné, A. and Liedholm, H. (2001). Survival after initial hospitalisation for heart failure: a multilevel analysis of patients in Swedish acute care hospitals. *Journal of Epidemiology and Community Health*, **55**, 323–9.

Merlo, J. (2003). Multilevel analytical approaches in social epidemiology: measures of health variation compared with traditional measures of association. *Journal of Epidemiology and Community Health*, **57**, 550–2.

Moerbeek, M., Breukelen van, G.J.P. and Berger, M.P.F. (2000). Design issues for multilevel experiments. *Journal of Educational and Behavioral Statistics*, **25**, 271–84.

Moerbeek, M., van Breukelen, G.J.P. and Berger, M.P.F. (2001). Optimal experimental designs for multilevel logistic models. *The Statistician*, **50**, 17–30.

Moerbeek, M., van Breukelen, G.J.P. and Berger, M.P.F. (2003a). A comparison between traditional methods and multilevel regression for the analysis of multicenter intervention studies. *Journal of Clinical Epidemiology*, **56**, 341–50.

Moerbeek, M., van Breukelen, G.J.P. and Berger, M.P.F. (2003b). A comparison of estimation methods for multilevel logistic models. *Computational Statistics*, **18**, 19–37.

Moerbeek, M., van Breukelen, G.J.P., Ausems, M. and Berger, M.P.F. (2003c). Optimal sample sizes in experimental designs with individuals nested within clusters. *Understanding Statistics*, **2**, 151–75.

Moerbeek, M. (2004). The consequence of ignoring a level of nesting in multilevel analysis. *Multivariate Behavioral Research*, **39**, 129–49.

Nelder, J.A. and Lee, Y. (1992). Likelihood, quasi-likelihood and pseudo-likelihood: some comparisons. *Journal of the Royal Statistical Society, B*, **54**, 273–84.

Neuhaus, J.M., Kalbfleisch, J.D. and Hauck, W.W. (1991). A comparison of cluster-specific and population-averaged approaches for analyzing correlated binary data. *International Statistical Reviews*, **59**, 25–36.

Neuhaus, J.M. and Lesparance, M.L. (1996). Estimation efficiency in a binary mixed-effects model setting. *Biometrika*, **83**, 441–6.

Neuhaus, J.M. and Kalbfleisch, J.D. (1998). Between- and within-cluster covariate effects in the analysis of clustered data. *Biometrics*, **54**, 638–45.

Nuttall, D.L., Goldstein, H., Prosser, R. and Rasbash, J. (1989). Differential school effectiveness. *International Journal of Educational Research*, **13**, 769–76.

O'Connor, B.P. (2004). SPSS and SAS programming for addressing interdependence and basic levels-of-analysis issues in psychological data. *Behavior Research Methods, Instruments, and Computers*, **36**, 17–28.

Omar, R.Z., Wright, E.M., Turner, R.M. and Thompson, S.G. (1999). Analyzing repeated measurements data: a practical comparison of methods. *Statistics in Medicine*, **18**, 1587–603.

Omar, R.Z. and Thompson, S.G. (2000). Analysis of a cluster randomised trial with binary outcome data using a multilevel model. *Statistics in Medicine*, **19**, 2675–88.

Opdenakker, M.-C. and Damme, van, J. (2000). The importance of identifying levels in multilevel analysis: an illustration of the effects of ignoring the top or intermediate levels in school effectiveness research. *School Effectiveness and School Improvement*, **11**, 103–30.

Pan, H.Q. and Goldstein, H. (1997). Multilevel models for longitudinal growth norms. *Statistics in Medicine*, **16**, 2665–78.

Pinheiro, J.C. and Bates, D.M. (2000). *Mixed-effects Models in S and S-PLUS*. New York: Springer-Verlag.

Plewis, I. (1991). Using multilevel models to link educational progress with curriculum coverage. In *Schools, Classrooms and Pupils. International Studies of Schooling from a Multilevel Perspective*, eds. S.W. Raudenbush, and J.D. Willms, San Diego: Academic Press.

Plewis, I. (1996). Statistical methods for understanding cognitive growth: a review, a synthesis and an application. *British Journal of Mathematical Statistical Psychology*, **49**, 25–42.

Plewis, I. and Hurry, J. (1998). A multilevel perspective on the design and analysis of intervention studies. *Educational Research and Evaluation*, **4**, 13–26.

Plewis, I. (2000). Evaluating educational interventions using multilevel growth curves: the case of reading recovery. *Educational Research and Evaluation*, **6**, 83–101.

R Development Core Team (2004). *R: A Language and Environment for Statistical Computing*. Vienna, Austria: R Foundation for Statistical Computing URL http://www.R-project.org.

Rabe-Hesketh, S. and Pickles, A. (1999). Generalised linear latent and mixed models. In *Proceedings of the 14th International Workshop on Statistical Modelling*, eds. H. Friedl, A. Bughold and G. Kauermann, pp. 332–9. Graz, Austria.

Rabe-Hesketh, S., Pickles, A. and Taylor, C. (2000). sg129: generalized linear latent and mixed models. *Stata Technical Bulletin*, **53**, 47–57.

Rabe-Hesketh, S. and Skrondal, A. (2001a). Parameterization of multivariate random effects models for categorical data. *Biometrics*, **57**, 1256–64.

Rabe-Hesketh, S., Pickles, A. and Skrondal, A. (2001b). *GLAMM Manual Technical Report 2001/01*. Department of Biostatistics and Computing, Institute of Psychiatry, King's college, University of London.

Rabe-Hesketh, S., Pickles, A. and Skrondal, A. (2001c). GLLAMM: A class of models and a Stata program. *Multilevel Modelling Newsletter*, 13, 17–23.

Rabe-Hesketh, S., Skrondal, A. and Pickles, A. (2002). Reliable estimation of generalized linear mixed models using adaptive quadrature. *The Stata Journal*, 2, 1–21.

Rabe-Hesketh, S., and Everitt, B.S. (2004). *Handbook of Statistical Analysis Using Stata*, 3rd edition. Boca Raton, FL: Chapman & Hall/CRC.

Rabe-Hesketh, S., Skrondal, A. and Pickles A. (2004). *GLLAMM Manual*. U.C. Berekely Division of Biostatistics Working Paper Series, paper 160,

URL http://www.bepres.com/ucbbiostat/paper160.

Rasbash, J., Browne, W., Goldstein, H., Yang, M., Plewis, I., Healy, M., Woodhouse, G. and Draper, D. (1999). *A User's Guide to MLwiN*, 2nd edition. London: Institute of Education.

Rasbash, J., Steele, F., Browne, W. and Prosser, B. (2003). *A User's Guide to MlwiN. Version 2.0*. London, UK: Centre for Multilevel Modelling, Institute of Education, University of London.

Raudenbush, S.W., Bryk, A.S., Cheong, Y.F. and Congdon, R. (2001). *HML5, Hierarchical Linear and Nonlinear Modelling*. SSI, Lincolnwood.

Raudenbush, S.W. and Bryk, A.S. (2002). *Hierarchical Linear Models. Applications and Data Analysis Methods*. Thousand Oaks: Sage Publications.

Reise, S.P. and Duan, N. (2003). *Multilevel Modelling Methodological Advances, Issues, and Applications*. Mahwah, NJ: Lawrence Erlbaum Associates.

Rice, N. and Leyland, A. (1996). Multilevel models: applications to health data. *Journal of Health Services Research Policy*, 1, 154–64.

Rochon, J. (1996). Analyzing bivariate repeated measures for discrete and continuous outcome variables. *Biometrics*, 52, 740–50.

Rodriguez, G. and Goldman, N. (1995). An assessment of estimation procedures for multilevel models with binary responses. *Journal of the Royal Statistical Association*, 158, 73–89.

Rodriguez, G. and Goldman, N. (1997). Multilevel models with binary response: a comparison of estimation procedures. *Journal of the Royal Statistical Society, A*, 158, 73–89.

Rodriguez, G. and Goldman, N. (2001). Improved estimation procedures for multilevel models with binary responses: a case study. *Journal of the Royal Statistical Association*, 164, 339–55.

Rubin, D.B. (1987). *Multiple imputation for nonresponse in surveys*. New York: John Wiley & Sons.

Rubin, D.B. (1996). Multiple imputation after 18+ years. *Journal of the American Statistical Association*, 91, 473–89.

SAS Institute Inc. (1997). *SAS/STAT Software: Changes and Enhancements Through Release 6.12*. Cary. NC.

Sastry, N. (1997). A nested frailty model for survival data, with an application to the study of child survival in northeast Brazil. *Journal of the American Statistical Association*, 92, 426–35.

Schafer, J.L. (1997). *Analysis of Incomplete Multivariate Data*. New York: Chapman & Hall.

Schafer, J.L. (1999). Multiple imputation: a primer. *Statistical Methods in Medical Research*, **8**, 3–15.

Schieke, T.H. and Jensen, T.K. (1997). A discrete survival model with random effects: an application to time to pregnancy. *Biometrics*, **53**, 318–29.

Schwarz, G. (1978). Estimating the dimensions of a model. *Annals of Statistics*, **6**, 461–4.

Shih, W.J. and Quan, H. (1997). Testing for treatment differences with dropouts present in clinical trials – a composite approach. *Statistics in Medicine*, **16**, 1225–39.

Skrondal, A. and Rabe-Hesketh, S. (2003a). Multilevel logistic regression for polytomous data and rankings. *Psychometrika*, **68**, 267–87.

Skrondal, A. and Rabe-Hesketh, S. (2003b). Some applications of generalized latent and mixed models in epidemiology. Repeated measures, measurement error and multilevel modelling. *Norwegian Journal of Epidemiology*, **13**, 265–78.

Skrondal, A. and Rabe-Hesketh, S. (2004). *Generalized Latent Variable Modeling: Multi-level, Longitudinal and Structural Equation Models*. Boca Raton, FL: Chapman & Hall/CRC Press.

Snijders, T.A.B. and Bosker, R.J. (1993). Standard errors and sample sizes for two-level research. *Journal of Educational Statistics*, **18**, 237–59.

Snijders, T.A.B. and Bosker, R.J. (1999). *Multilevel Analysis. An Introduction to Basic and Advanced Multilevel Modelling*. London: Sage Publications.

Stata Corporation. (1999). *Stata Statistical Software: Release 6*. College Station, Texas, USA: Stata Press.

Stata Reference Manual. (2001). *Release 7*. College Station, Texas: Stata Press.

Stoel, R.D. (2003). *Issues in growth curve modeling (PhD-thesis)*. Amsterdam, The Netherlands: T-T Pubikaties.

Ten Have, T.R. (1996). A mixed effects model for multivariate ordinal response data including correlated discrete failure times with ordinal responses. *Biometrics*, **52**, 473–91.

Thompson, A.M., Baxter-Jones, A.D.G., Mirwald, R.L. and Bailey, D.A. (2003). Comparison of physical activity levels in male and female children using chronological and biological ages. *Medicine and Science in Sports and Exercise*, **35**, 1684–90.

Thum, Y.M. (1997). Hierarchical linear models for multivariate outcomes. *Journal of Educational and Behavioural Statistics*, **22**, 77–108.

Tranmer, M. and Steel, D.G. (2001). Ignoring a level in a multilevel model: evidence from UK census data. *Environment and Planning A*, **33**, 941–8.

Turner, R.M., Omar, R.Z. and Thompson, S.G. (2001). Bayesian methods of analysis for cluster randomised trials with binary outcome data. *Statistics in Medicine*, **20**, 453–72.

Twisk, J.W.R. and Vente W. de. (2002). Attrition in longitudinal studies. How to deal with missing data. *Journal of Clinical Epidemiology*, **55**, 329–337.

Twisk, J.W.R. (2003). *Applied Longitudinal Data Analysis for Epidemiology. A Practical Guide*. Cambridge: Cambridge University Press.

Twisk, J.W.R. and Proper, K. (2004). Evaluation of the results of a randomized controlled trial: how to define changes between baseline and follow-up. *Journal of Clinical Epidemiology*, **57**, 223–28.

Twisk, J.W.R. (2004). Longitudinal data analysis: a comparison between generalized estimating equations and random coefficient analysis. *European Journal of Epidemiology*, **19**, 769–76.

Vaida, F. and Xu, R. (2001). Proportional hazards model with random effects. *Statistics in Medicine*, **20**, 3309–24.

Venables, W.N. and Ripley, B.D. (2002). *Modern applied statistics with S*, 4th edition. New York: Springer.

Venables, W.N. and Ripley, B.D. (2000), *S Programming*. New York: Springer.

Wampold, B.E. and Serlin, R.C. (2000). The consequence of ignoring a nested factor on measures of effect size in analysis of variance. *Psychological Methods*, **5**, 425–33.

Woodhouse, G. and Goldstein, H. (1989). Educational performance indicators and LEA league tables. *Oxford Review of Education*, **14**, 301–19.

Wolfinger, R., Tobias, R. and Sall, J. (1994). Computing Gaussian likelihoods and their derivates for general linear mixed models. *SIAM Journal of Scientific Computation*, **15**, 1294–310.

Xu, J. and Zeger, S.L. (2001). Joint analysis of longitudinal data comprising repeated measures and times to events. *Journal of the Royal Statistical Society, C*, **50**, 375–88.

Yang, M. (1997). Multilevel models for multiple category responses by *MLn* simulation. *Multilevel Modelling Newsletter*, **9**, 9–15.

Yang, M., Rasbash, J., Goldstein, H. and Barbosa, M. (1999). *MLwiN macros for advanced multilevel modelling (version 2.0)*. London: Institute of Education, Centre for multilevel modelling.

Yau, K.K.W. (2001). Multilevel models for survival analysis with random effects. *Biometrics*, **57**, 96–102.

Zeger, S.L. and Liang, K.-Y. (1986). Longitudinal data analysis for discrete and continuous outcomes. *Biometrics*. **42**, 121–30.

Zeger, S.L. and Liang, K.-Y. (1992). An overview of methods for the analysis of longitudinal data. *Statistics in Medicine*, **11**, 1825–39.

Index